ABC OF CLINICAL GENETICS

ABC OF CLINICAL GENETICS

HELEN M KINGSTON
Consultant clinical geneticist
St Mary's Hospital, Manchester

Articles published in
the *British Medical Journal*

Published by the British Medical Association
Tavistock Square, London WC1H 9JR

First published 1989

British Library Cataloguing in Publication Data

Kingston, Helen M
    ABC of clinical genetics
    1. Man. Genetics. Medical aspects
    I. Title   II. British Medical Journal
    616'.042

ISBN 0-7279-0263-6

Printed in Great Britain by Jolly & Barber Ltd, Rugby
Typesetting by Bedford Typesetters Ltd, Bedford

Contents

ACKNOWLEDGMENTS

In writing this series I have been greatly influenced by my former teachers of clinical genetics, particularly Professors Peter Harper and Michael Laurence, to whom I am grateful. I have benefited from helpful suggestions on the text from Professor Rodney Harris, Dr Dian Donnai, and Dr Andrew Read of St Mary's Hospital, and thank many colleagues in Manchester who have generously provided illustrations for the series, and Margaret Trickey for typing the original manuscripts.

HMK

CLINICAL GENETIC SERVICES

Genetic disease

Type of genetic disease

Single gene (mendelian)	Numerous though individually rare Clear pattern of inheritance High risk to relatives
Multifactorial	Common disorders No clear pattern of inheritance Low or moderate risk to relatives
Chromosomal	Mostly rare No clear pattern of inheritance Usually low risk to relatives
Somatic mutation	Accounts for mosaicism Cause of neoplasia

Genetic disorders place considerable health and economic burdens not only on affected people and their families but also on the community. As more environmental diseases are successfully controlled those that are wholly or partly genetically determined are becoming more important.

Despite a general fall in perinatal mortality rate the incidence of lethal malformations in newborn infants remains constant. Between 2-5% of all liveborn infants have genetic disorders or congenital malformations. These disorders have been estimated to account for one third of admissions to paediatric wards, and they contribute appreciably to paediatric mortality. Many common diseases in adult life also have a considerable genetic predisposition, including coronary heart disease, diabetes, and cancer.

Prevalence of genetic disease

Type of genetic disease	Estimated prevalence per 1000 population
Single gene:	
Autosomal dominant	2-10
Autosomal recessive	2
X linked recessive	1-2
Chromosomal abnormalities	6-7
Common disorders with appreciable genetic component	7-10
Congenital malformations	20
Total	38-51

Though diseases of wholly genetic origin are often individually rare, they are numerous and therefore important. Genetic disorders are incurable and often severe. A few are amenable to treatment, but most are not, so that emphasis is often placed on prevention of either recurrence within an affected family or complications in a person who is already affected.

Increasing awareness, both within the medical profession and in the general population, of the genetic contribution to disease has led to an increasing demand for clinical genetic services. Some aspects of genetics are well established and do not require referral to a specialised genetics clinic—for example, the provision of amniocentesis to exclude Down's syndrome in pregnancies at risk because of advanced maternal age. Other aspects are less well understood by non-geneticists—for example, the role of molecular biology in clinical practice, which is an area of rapidly advancing technology requiring the specialised facilities of a genetics centre.

Aims of genetic counselling

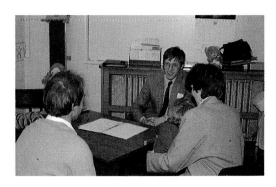

Genetic counselling covers more than estimating risks and extends beyond the person who presents to the whole family in changing situations over many years. The role of clinical geneticists is to establish an accurate diagnosis on which to base counselling and then to provide information about prognosis and follow up, the risk of developing or transmitting the disorder, and the ways in which this may be prevented or ameliorated. Throughout, the family require support in adjusting to the implications of genetic disease and the consequent decisions that have to be made.

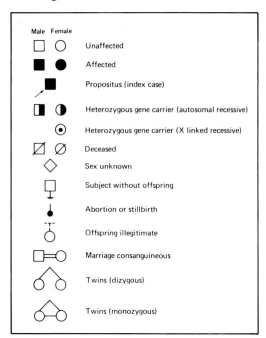

Diagnosis

An accurate diagnosis is the first essential requirement for genetic counselling. This may not always be straightforward as genetic disease is often variable in its presentation and different members of a family with the same disorder may present to different specialties with diverse manifestations of the condition. Conversely, disorders which are clinically similar may follow different inheritance patterns in different families.

The person requesting genetic counselling may not be the one affected, and the diagnosis may need to be confirmed by examining the affected relative or reviewing their hospital records.

Without a defined diagnosis appropriate genetic advice may be given if the pattern of affected subjects within a family points to a particular mode of inheritance.

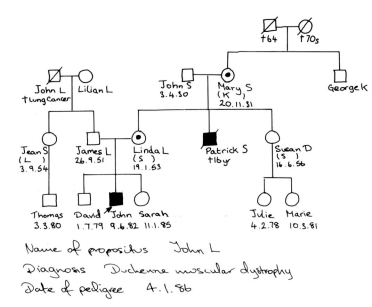

Name of propositus   John L
Diagnosis   Duchenne muscular dystrophy
Date of pedigree   4.1.86

Drawing a pedigree

Constructing a family tree is the best way to record genetic information. The main symbols used are shown in the upper box. It is important to record full names (including maiden names) and dates of birth on the pedigree. Specific questions should be asked about abortions, stillbirths, infant deaths, multiple marriages, and consanguinity as this information may not always be volunteered. It is also useful to record details of the medical care of relevant family members.

Common reasons for referral to a genetics clinic

Genetic disease diagnosed, counselling requested

Testing carrier state of family members for mendelian disorders

Investigation and diagnosis of possible genetic disease

Diagnosis of mental handicap or physical abnormality

Diagnosis of malformation in neonates or stillbirths

Genetic investigation of recurrent pregnancy loss

Genetic management of high risk pregnancies

Interpretation of abnormal prenatal tests

Estimation of risk

Estimation of genetic risk depends on the pattern of inheritance of a disorder and applies both to the risk of developing and of transmitting a particular disorder. In some disorders specific tests to identify carriers are available.

Mendelian disorders due to mutant genes generally carry high risks of recurrence whereas chromosomal disorders generally have low risks. For many common conditions there is no clearly defined pattern of inheritance, and empirical figures for the risk of recurrence are given, based on information derived from family studies.

Transmitting information

Interpretation of risk varies depending on the severity of the disorder, its prognosis, and the availability of treatment or palliation. All of these aspects need to be discussed with the family.

The risk of transmitting a disorder, the severity of the disorder, and the availability of prenatal diagnosis all influence the decisions of couples about pregnancy, as do their moral and religious convictions. Contraception or sterilisation may be considered, and alternative options may include insemination by a donor, ovum donation, or adoption.

It is important that the counselling process is not directive and that couples can reach their own decisions armed with the necessary information.

Psychological aspects

The diagnosis of genetic disease causes considerable emotional stress, and to be effective the counselling process must provide psychological support in addition to information. Recognition of the impact of genetic disease and the various stages of the process of coping allows counselling to be pursued at an appropriate pace for each couple. Some knowledge of the couples' educational, social, and religious backgrounds is important as these influence their reactions and decision making.

Counselling must be unhurried and undertaken in a quiet environment. The counsellor needs to spend sufficient time with the couple to establish mutual rapport, so that personal feelings can be freely discussed and questions asked and dealt with sensitively; several counselling sessions, either in the clinic or at the patient's home may be necessary to achieve this.

Main users of clinical genetic services
Paediatricians
Obstetricians
Other hospital specialists
General practitioners
Community child health services
Others (self referrals, adoption services)

Organisation of clinical services

Medical staff	Consultant clinicial geneticists
	Senior registrar
	Research registrar
	Clinical assistants or clinical medical officers
Field workers	Genetic associates (scientific officers or counsellors)
	Specialist health visitors
	Social workers
	Phlebotomist
Clerical staff	

Departments of clinical genetics tend to be based regionally in main teaching centres and often have academic as well as NHS staff. The clinical team includes various health care professionals.

Associated laboratory services

Specialist laboratory services form an integral part in providing clinical genetic services. The laboratories are usually based in regional or supraregional centres and provide services in biochemical genetics, cytogenetics, and molecular genetics.

Genetic registers

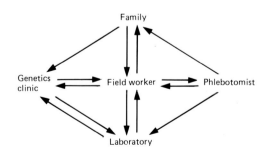

Clinical use of genetic registers is aimed primarily at ascertaining as completely as possible all people at risk of developing or transmitting a particular disorder so that appropriate counselling can be offered. A register approach permits long term follow up of family members, which is important for children at risk, who will not need investigation or counselling for many years. Registers are particularly useful for disorders that are amenable to DNA analysis in which advances are of clinical importance and families need regular counselling with new information. Disorders suited to a register approach include dominant disorders with late onset, such as Huntington's chorea and myotonic dystrophy, and X linked disorders, such as Duchenne and Becker's muscular dystrophy. Registers can also provide data on the incidence and natural course of diseases and the effect of counselling and preventive programmes.

Genetic registers are held on computer and are subject to the Data Protection Act. No one is included in a register without having given informed consent.

MENDELIAN INHERITANCE

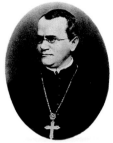

Gregor Mendel 1822-84

Disorders caused by a defect in a single gene follow the patterns of inheritance described by Mendel. Individual disorders of this type are often rare but are important because they are numerous (over 4000 single gene traits have been listed[1]). Risks within an affected family are usually high and are calculated by knowing the mode of inheritance and details of the family pedigree.

Autosomal dominant disorders

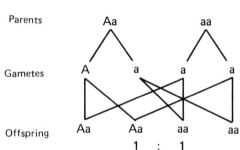

Autosomal dominant disorders affect both males and females and can often be traced through many generations of a family. Affected people are heterozygous for the abnormal allele and transmit the gene for the disease to half their offspring, whether male or female. The disorder is not transmitted by family members who are unaffected themselves. Estimation of risk is therefore apparently simple, but in practice several factors may cause difficulties in counselling families.

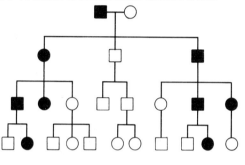

Parents	Aa		aa	
Gametes	A	a	a	a
Offspring	Aa	Aa	aa	aa
	1	:	1	

Firstly, the age of onset of a disorder may be variable and people with a defective gene, who are destined to become affected, may remain without signs or symptoms well into adult life. Young people at risk may not know whether they have inherited the disorder and will transmit it to their children, at a time when they are planning their own families. Detection of people carrying the mutant gene before symptoms become apparent may therefore be important in conditions such as Huntington's chorea and myotonic dystrophy.

The severity of many dominant conditions also varies considerably among affected members within a family. The likely severity in any affected offspring is difficult to predict, and a mildly affected parent may have a severely affected child, as illustrated by tuberous sclerosis, in which a parent with only skin manifestations of the disorder may have an affected child with infantile spasms and severe mental retardation.

New mutation may account for the presence of a dominant disorder in a subject who does not have a family history of the disease. When a disorder arises by new mutation the risk of recurrence in future pregnancies for the mother of the affected child is negligible. Care must be

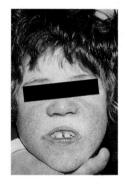

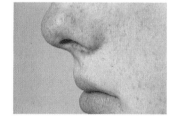

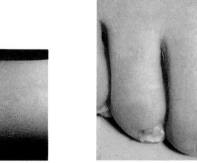

Tuberous sclerosis. Top left: severely affected boy with fits and mental retardation; top right: adenoma sebaceum; bottom left: ash leaf depigmentation; bottom right: periungal fibroma.

Examples of autosomal dominant disorders

Achondroplasia	Huntington's chorea
Acute intermittent porphyria	Myotonic dystrophy
Adult polycystic kidney disease	Noonan's syndrome
Alzheimer's disease (some cases)	Neurofibromatosis
Epidermolysis bullosa (some forms)	Osteogenesis imperfecta (some forms)
Facioscapulohumeral dystrophy	Polyposis coli
Familial hypercholesterolaemia	Tuberous sclerosis

taken to exclude a mild form of the condition in one or other parent before giving this reassurance. New mutation accounts for most cases of achondroplasia, a condition that can be easily excluded in the parents. On the other hand, neurofibromatosis may arise by new mutation or be present in mild form in one parent. In dominant conditions an apparently normal parent may occasionally carry a germline mutation; this is associated with a considerable risk of recurrence. A dominant disorder in a person with a negative family history may alternatively indicate non-paternity.

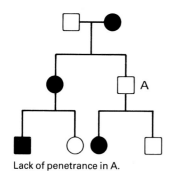

Lack of penetrance in A.

A few dominant disorders show lack of penetrance—that is, a person who inherits the gene does not develop the disorder. In this case people who are not affected cannot be completely reassured that they will not transmit the disorder to their children. The risk is, however, fairly low, not exceeding 10%, because when penetrance is high an unaffected person is unlikely to be a gene carrier, and when it is low the chance of a gene carrier developing the disorder is correspondingly small.

Non-genetic factors may also influence the expression of dominant genes—for example, diet in hypercholesterolaemia and drugs in porphyria.

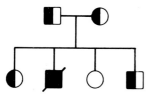

■	Homozygous affected
◧	Heterozygous affected

Homozygosity for a dominant disorder.

Homozygosity for dominant genes is uncommon, unless two people with the same disorder marry. This may happen preferentially with certain conditions, such as achondroplasia. Homozygous achondroplasia is a lethal condition and the risks for offspring are therefore: 25% homozygous affected (lethal); 50% heterozygous affected; 25% homozygous normal. Thus two out of three living children will be affected.

Autosomal recessive disorders

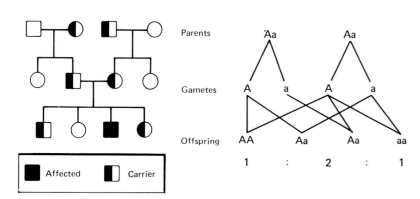

Parents

Gametes

Offspring

Aa		Aa	
A a		A a	
AA	Aa	Aa	aa
1	: 2	:	1

■ Affected	◧ Carrier

Autosomal recessive disorders occur in a person whose healthy parents both carry the same recessive gene. The risk of recurrence for future offspring of such parents is 25%. Unlike autosomal dominant disorders there is generally no family history. Although the defective gene may be passed from generation to generation, the disorder generally only appears within a single sibship—that is, within one group of brothers and sisters.

In northern Europeans the commonest autosomal recessive disorder is cystic fibrosis, and about one in 20 people in the population is a carrier.

Consanguinity increases the risk of a recessive disorder because both parents are more likely to carry the same defective gene, which has been inherited from a common ancestor. The rarer the condition the more likely it is that the parents were related before marriage. Overall, the increased risk to parents who are first cousins of having a child with severe abnormalities is fairly low (3% above the risk in the general population), and this includes the risk of autosomal recessive disorders.

The offspring of an affected person will be healthy heterozygotes and can be affected only if the other parent is also a gene carrier. This is unlikely except in consanguineous marriages or in ethnic groups in which particular genes are common.

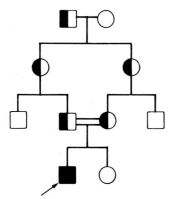

Consanguinity and autosomal recessive inheritance.

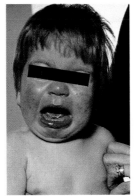

Hurler's syndrome: coarsening of facial features.

Mendelian inheritance

Examples of autosomal recessive disorders

Congenital adrenal hyperplasia	Homocystinuria
Cystic fibrosis	Hurler's syndrome (mucopolysaccharidosis I)
Deafness (some forms)	Laurence-Moon-Biedl syndrome
Diastrophic dwarfism	Occulocutaneous albinism
Epidermolysis bullosa (some forms)	Phenylketonuria
Friedreich's ataxia	Sickle cell disease
Galactosaemia	Tay-Sachs disease
Haemochromatosis	Thalassaemia

Autosomal recessive disorders are commonly severe, and many of the recognised inborn errors of metabolism follow this type of inheritance. Many complex malformation syndromes are also due to autosomal recessive genes, and their recognition is important in the first affected child in a family because of the 25% risk of recurrence. Prenatal diagnosis for recessive disorders may be possible by performing biochemical assays, DNA analysis, or looking for structural abnormalities in the fetus.

X linked recessive disorders

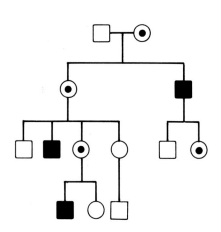

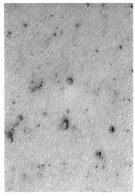

Angiokeratoma in Fabry's disease.

In X linked recessive conditions only males are affected and the disorder is transmitted through healthy female carriers. Occasionally a heterozygous female may show some features of the condition.

A female carrier will transmit the disorder to half her sons, and half her daughters will be carriers. All the daughters of an affected male are obligate carriers whereas none of the sons are affected. X linked recessive disorders cannot be transmitted by a healthy male. Many X linked recessive disorders are severe or lethal during early life, so that the affected males do not reproduce.

Examples of X linked disorders

Recessive

Anhidrotic ectodermal dysplasia	Haemophilia A, B
Becker's muscular dystrophy	Hunter's syndrome (mucopolysaccharidosis II)
Colour blindness	Lesch-Nyhan syndrome
Duchenne muscular dystrophy	Menkes's syndrome
Fabry's disease	Mental retardation with or without fragile site
Glucose-6-phosphate dehydrogenase deficiency	Occular albinism

Dominant

Incontinentia pigmenti	Rickets resistant to vitamin D
Orofaciodigital syndrome	

An X linked recessive condition should be considered when the family history indicates affected males in different generations of the family. Family history is, however, not always positive as new mutations are fairly common.

Identifying female gene carriers in the family requires interpretation of the family pedigree and the results of specific tests to identify the carriers.

X linked dominant disorders

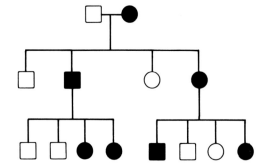

An X linked dominant gene will give rise to a disorder in both hemizygous males and heterozygous females. The gene is transmitted in families in the same way as X linked recessive genes, giving rise to an excess of affected females. In some disorders the condition is lethal in hemizygous males. In this case there will be fewer males than expected in the family, all of whom will be healthy, and an excess of females, half of whom will be affected.

Y linked disorders

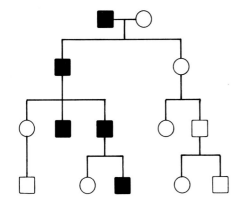

In Y linked disorders only males are affected, with transmission being directly from father to son with the Y chromosome. This pattern of inheritance has been suggested for such conditions as porcupine skin, hairy ears, and webbed toes. In most conditions in which Y linked inheritance has been postulated the actual mode of inheritance is probably autosomal dominant, with other factors causing sex limitation.

Cytoplasmic inheritance

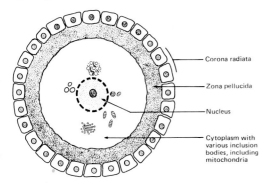

Diagrammatic representation of human egg.

Unlike sperm, the egg contains cytoplasm as well as a nucleus. Certain characteristics in the fetus are probably influenced or wholly determined by cytoplasmic elements including biochemical factors and mitochondrial DNA, and these would always be maternally derived. Although not proved, cytoplasmic factors may account for the maternal transmission of the congenital form of myotonic dystrophy and the preponderance of paternal transmission in Huntington's chorea of juvenile onset, as well as the transient myasthenia seen in the offspring of mothers with myasthenia gravis. Mutations in mitochondrial DNA have been reported in Leber's optic atrophy, which is exclusively maternally transmitted, and in certain mitochondrial myopathies, some types of which also show maternal inheritance.

1 McKusick VA. *Mendelian inheritance in man. Catalogs of autosomal dominant, autosomal recessive and X-linked phenotypes.* 8th ed. Baltimore: John Hopkins, 1988.

The illustrations of tuberous sclerosis were reproduced by kind permission of Professor P S Harper, Institute of Medical Genetics for Wales, Cardiff.

ESTIMATION OF RISK

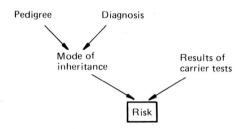

This chapter gives some examples of the risk of developing or transmitting a mendelian disorder. The mathematical risk calculated from data on a pedigree may often be modied by additional information from specific tests to detect carriers. Risk can be expressed as either a percentage or a fraction.

Autosomal dominant disorders

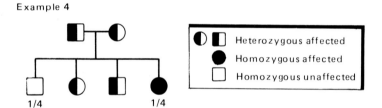

Example 1.

B Aged 30, risk = 1/2

C Aged 8, risk = 1/4

Example 2.

B Aged 60, risk = 1/10

C Aged 30, risk = 1/20

Example 3.

B † Aged 30

C Aged 30, risk = 1/4

The 50% risk of developing a condition for the offspring of an affected person may be modified by age in disorders whose onset is in adult life, such as Huntington's chorea. In examples 1 and 2 the risk to person B of developing Huntington's chorea is still 50% at age 30 years, but by the age of 60 the residual risk to a healthy person has fallen to about 10%. The risk to person C therefore falls from 25% in example 1 to 5% in example 2. In example 3 the risk for C cannot be reduced below 25% because parent B, although clinically unaffected, died aged 30 while still at 50% risk.

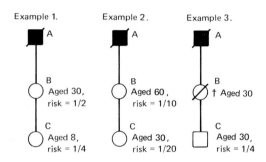

Example 4

◑ ◐	Heterozygous affected
●	Homozygous affected
☐	Homozygous unaffected

1/4 ... 1/4

When both parents have the same autosomal dominant disorder, the risk to the offspring will be high (example 4). Only one in four children will be unaffected, and one in four will be homozygous for the mutant gene, which may cause severe disease, as in familial hypercholesterolaemia or achondroplasia.

Example 5

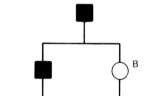

Person	Risk of having inherited gene (%)	Risk of developing disorder (%)
A	50	40
C	8	6-7

Reduced penetrance also modifies simple autosomal dominant risk. Example 5 shows the risks for a disorder with 80% penetrance in which only 80% of gene carriers develop the disorder. Although clinically unaffected, person B may still carry the mutant gene, and there is therefore a fairly small risk of her child developing the disorder.

Autosomal recessive disorders

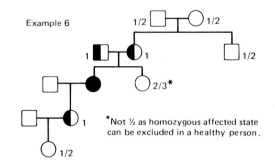

Example 6

*Not ½ as homozygous affected state can be excluded in a healthy person.

Recurrence of autosomal recessive disorders generally only occurs within a particular sibship. Many members of the family, however, may be gene carriers, the risks of which are shown in example 6.

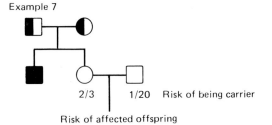

Example 7

2/3   1/20   Risk of being carrier

Risk of affected offspring

2/3 x 1/20 x 1/4 = 1/120

The chance of a healthy sibling having affected children is low. The actual risk depends on the frequency of the gene in the general population. The risk for cystic fibrosis is shown in example 7. (In the general population about one in 20 people are gene carriers.)

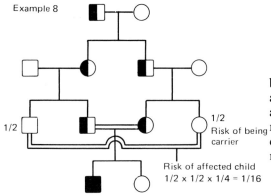

Example 8

1/2

1/2   Risk of being carrier

Risk of affected child
1/2 x 1/2 x 1/4 = 1/16

When there is a tradition of consanguinity more than one marriage may be arranged between two families. If a consanguineous couple have a child affected by an autosomal recessive condition other family marriages may also be at risk of having affected offspring, as in example 8. The risk may not be high enough to prevent further planned marriages taking place, but if carrier state can be determined by specific tests this will help the families to make decisions and reassure the relatives who are not carriers.

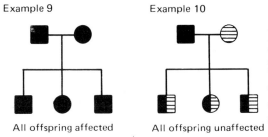

Example 9   Example 10

All offspring affected   All offspring unaffected

When both parents are affected by a recessive condition such as deafness the risks to the offspring will depend on whether the parents are homozygous for allelic or non-allelic genes as some autosomal recessive disorders can be caused by different genes at separate loci. In example 9 both parents have the same form of recessive deafness and all their children will be affected. In example 10 the parents have different forms of recessive deafness due to genes at different loci. Their offspring will be heterozygous at both loci and therefore unaffected.

X linked recessive disorders

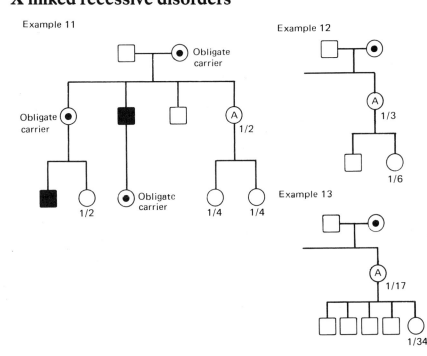

Example 11

Obligate carrier

Obligate carrier

A 1/2

Obligate carrier

1/2   1/4   1/4

Example 12

A 1/3

1/6

Example 13

A 1/17

1/34

Calculation of risks in X linked recessive disorders is often complex, and the following examples illustrate some basic concepts without details of method. Referral to a specialist genetic centre is usually indicated for calculating carrier state, which depends on pedigree structure and results of specific tests. In families with X linked recessive disorders many female relatives are at risk of being carriers, as in example 11.

If the female relative A at risk in example 11 has any healthy sons this will reduce her risk to the values shown in examples 12 and 13.

Estimation of risk

Example 14

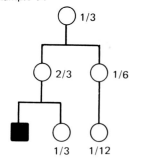
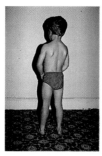
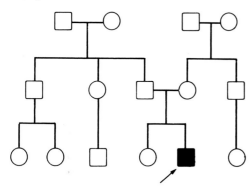

In lethal X linked recessive disorders new mutations account for a third of all cases. A mother of an affected boy is therefore not always a carrier. Carrier risks in families in which there is an isolated case of such a disorder (for example, Duchenne muscular dystrophy) are shown in example 14. These risks would again be modified by the presence of any unaffected males in the pedigree as well as by the results of specific tests to detect carriers.

Winging of scapulae, exaggerated lumbar lordosis, and prominent calf muscles in boy with Duchenne muscular dystrophy.

Isolated cases

Example 15

Pedigrees showing only one affected person are the type most commonly encountered in clinical practice (example 15). Various causes must be considered, and counselling in this situation depends entirely on reaching an accurate diagnosis in the affected person.

Possible causes

- Non-genetic

- Autosomal dominant: new mutation, non-paternity, or (rarely) parental germline mutation

- Autosomal recessive

- X linked recessive. May represent new mutation or inheritance from carrier mother

- Polygenic (multifactorial). Risk of recurrence generally low

- Chromosomal. Recurrence depends on type of abnormality, but generally low

Example 16

Risk of recurrence
$7/10 \times 2/3 \times 1/4 \; \widehat{=} \; 1/9$

In example 16 calculation of the risk of recurrence after an isolated case of congenital deafness is based on the finding that when environmental causes are excluded 70% of cases are genetic, of which two thirds are autosomal recessive.

DETECTION OF CARRIERS

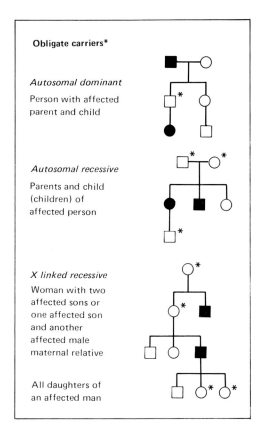

Obligate carriers*

Autosomal dominant
Person with affected parent and child

Autosomal recessive
Parents and child (children) of affected person

X linked recessive
Woman with two affected sons or one affected son and another affected male maternal relative

All daughters of an affected man

Identifying carriers of genetic disorders in families or populations at risk plays an important part in preventing genetic disease. A carrier is a healthy person who possesses the mutant gene for an inherited disorder in the heterozygous state. The term carrier is therefore restricted to people at risk of transmitting mendelian disorders and does not apply to parents whose children have chromosomal abnormalities or congenital malformations such as neural tube defect. An exception is that people who have balanced chromosomal translocations are referred to as carriers as the inheritance of balanced or unbalanced translocations follows mendelian principles.

In families in which there is a genetic disorder some members must be carriers because of the way in which the condition is inherited. These obligate carriers can be identified by drawing a family pedigree and do not require testing as their genetic state is not in doubt. Identification of obligate carriers is important not only for their counselling but also for defining a group in whom tests for carrier state can be evaluated. Knowledge is needed of the proportion of obligate carriers showing abnormalities on clinical examination or with specific investigations and of the age at which such abnormalities appear to assess the likelihood of carrier state in the other relatives.

In some disorders—for example, sickle cell disease—all carriers can be identified with certainty; in others—for example, tuberous sclerosis—only a proportion can be identified. In autosomal dominant and X linked recessive disorders parental carrier state may be particularly difficult to assess because of the additional possibilities of new mutation in the child or germline mosaicism in the parent.

Autosomal dominant disorders

Some autosomal dominant disorders amenable to carrier detection

Adult polycystic kidney disease

Familial hypercholesterolaemia

Huntington's chorea

Malignant hyperpyrexia

Myotonic dystrophy

Neurofibromatosis

Tuberous sclerosis

. von Hippel-Lindau disease

In autosomal dominant conditions most heterozygous subjects are clinically affected and testing for carrier state applies only to disorders that are either variable in their manifestations or have a late onset. Gene carriers in conditions such as tuberous sclerosis may be mildly affected but run the risk of having severely affected children whereas carriers in other disorders, such as Huntington's chorea, are destined to develop severe disease themselves.

Identifying symptomless gene carriers allows a couple to make informed decisions about having children, may indicate a need to avoid environmental triggers (as in porphyria), or may permit early treatment and prevention of complications (for example, in von Hippel-Lindau disease). Although testing for carrier state can have important benefits in conditions in which the prognosis is improved by early detection, presymptomatic diagnosis of severe disorders, such as Huntington's chorea, that are not amenable to treatment presents problems. Exclusion of carrier state is, however, equally important, removing anxiety about transmitting the condition to offspring and the need for long term follow up.

Detection of carriers
Autosomal recessive disorders

In autosomal recessive conditions carriers remain healthy. Occasionally, heterozygous subjects may show minor abnormalities, such as altered red cell morphology in sickle cell disease and mild anaemia in thalassaemia. Most inborn errors of metabolism follow autosomal recessive inheritance, and heterozygous subjects may show reduced activities of specific enzymes, which provides the basis for detecting carriers.

The parents of an affected child are obligate carriers, but testing may be appropriate for the healthy siblings of an affected person and their partner if the condition is fairly common. Testing may also be important for consanguineous couples with a positive family history of genetic disease. The main opportunity for preventing autosomal recessive disorders, however, depends on population screening programmes, which will identify couples at risk before the birth of an affected child within the family. Screening subgroups of the population at high risk has proved effective in Tay-Sachs disease and β thalassaemia and will be appropriate for cystic fibrosis once a reliable test is available.

X linked recessive disorders

Carrier detection in X linked recessive conditions is particularly important as these disorders are often severe and in an affected family many female relatives may be at risk of having affected sons, irrespective of whom they marry. Genetic counselling cannot be undertaken without accurate assessment of carrier state, and calculating the risk is often complex.

Obligate carriers do not always show abnormalities on biochemical testing because of lyonisation, a process by which one or other X chromosome in female embryos is randomly inactivated early in embryogenesis. The proportion of cells with the normal or mutant X chromosome remaining active varies and will influence detection of carrier state. Carriers with a high proportion of normal X chromosomes remaining active will show no abnormalities on biochemical testing. Conversely, carriers with a high proportion of mutant X chromosomes remaining active are more likely to show biochemical abnormalities and may occasionally develop signs and symptoms of the disorder. Females with symptoms are called manifesting carriers.

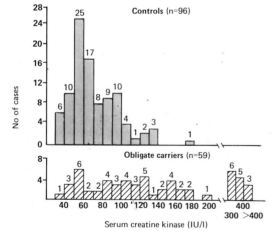

Overlapping ranges of serum creatine kinase activity in controls and obligate carriers of Becker's muscular dystrophy. (Ranges vary among laboratories.)

Biochemical tests designed to determine carrier state must be evaluated initially in obligate carriers identified from affected families. Only tests which give significantly different results in obligate carriers compared with controls will be useful in determining the genetic state of female subjects at risk. Because the ranges of values in obligate carriers and controls overlap considerably (for example serum creatine kinase activity in X linked muscular dystrophy) the results for possible carriers are expressed in relative terms as a likelihood ratio. With this type of test confirmation of carrier state is always easier than exclusion. In muscular dystrophy a high serum creatine kinase activity confirms the carrier state; a normal result reduces but does not eliminate the chance that a female is a carrier.

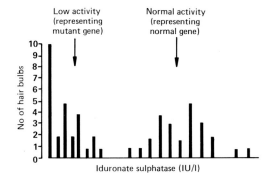

The problem of lyonisation can be largely overcome if biochemical tests can be performed on clonally derived cells; hair bulbs have been successfully used to detect carriers of Hunter's syndrome (mucopolysaccharidosis II). Carriers can be identified because they have two populations of hair bulbs, one with normal iduronate sulphatase activity, reflecting hair bulbs with the normal X chromosome remaining active, and the other with low enzyme activity, representing those with the mutant X chromosome remaining active.

Two populations of hair bulbs with low and normal activity of iduronate sulphatase, respectively, in female carrier of Hunter's syndrome.

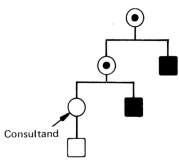

DNA analysis is not affected by lyonisation and is becoming an increasingly important method of detecting carriers as specific gene probes or linked probes become available. Such analysis is successful in defining low as well as high risk.

Calculation of the final probability of carrier state entails analysis of pedigree data with the results of one or more specific tests. The possibility of new mutation and gonadal mosaicism must be taken into account in sporadic cases. The calculation relies on Bayesian analysis, and computer programs are available for the complex analysis required in large families.

Information on consultand:

Prior risk = 50% (mother obligate carrier)

Risk modified by:

DNA analysis —reducing prior risk to 5%

One healthy son —reducing risk

Analysis of serum creatine kinase activity — giving probability of carrier state of 0·3

Risk after Bayesian calculation = 1%

Calculation of carrier risk in Duchenne muscular dystrophy.

Testing for carrier state

Various methods can be used to determine carrier state; those related directly to gene function discriminate better than those measuring functions further removed from the primary gene defect. Detection of an abnormality confirms the carrier state but its apparent absence does not guarantee normality.

Clinical signs

Careful examination for clinical signs may identify some carriers and is particularly important in autosomal dominant conditions in which the underlying biochemical basis of the disorder is unknown. In some X linked recessive disorders (especially those affecting the eye or skin) abnormalities may be detected in this way in female carriers. The absence of clinical signs does not exclude the carrier state.

Clinical examination can be supplemented with investigations such as physiological studies, microscopy, and radiology. In myotonic dystrophy, for example, carriers can usually be identified in early adult life before symptoms develop by a combination of clinical examination to detect myotonia and mild weakness of facial and sternomastoid muscles, slit lamp examination of the eyes to detect lens opacities, and electromyography to look for myotonic changes. Confirmation or exclusion of the carrier state is important for genetic counselling, especially for mildly affected women who have an appreciable risk of producing severely affected infants with the congenital form of myotonic dystrophy.

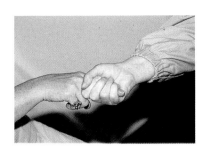

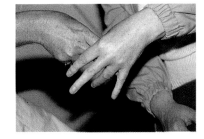

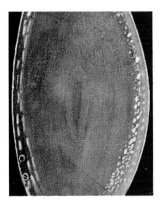

Clinical myotonia, lens opacities, and myotonic discharges on electromyography confirm carrier state in myotonic dystrophy.

Detection of carriers

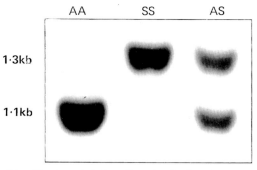

Identification of sickle cell carriers by Southern blot analysis of *Mst II* restriction fragments and β globin gene probe. (AA=Normal, AS=sickle cell trait, SS= sickle cell anaemia.)

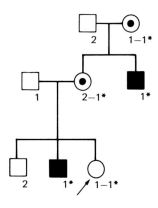

1,2 = DNA variants detected by probe linked to Duchenne muscular dystrophy gene on X chromosome

Prediction of carrier state by DNA analysis in Duchenne muscular dystrophy. Disease gene cosegregates with DNA variant 1*, predicting that consultand (↗) is a carrier.

Analysis of genes

DNA probes are becoming available for an increasing number of mendelian disorders and can be used to predict carrier state as well as for presymptomatic or prenatal diagnosis. Specific gene probes may sometimes permit direct identification of carriers (as in sickle cell disease), but family studies are usually required to track the abnormal gene through the family with linked DNA polymorphisms (variations).

Analysis of gene products

Biochemical identification of carriers may be possible when the gene product is known. This approach is used for inborn errors of metabolism due to enzyme deficiency as well as for disorders due to a defective structural protein, such as haemophilia and thalassaemia. Overlap between the ranges of values in heterozygous and normal people occurs even when the primary gene product can be analysed, and interpretation of results can be difficult.

Secondary biochemical abnormalities

When the gene product is not known or cannot be readily tested the identification of carriers may depend on detecting secondary biochemical abnormalities, such as raised serum creatine kinase activity in Duchenne and Becker's muscular dystrophies. The overlap between the ranges of values in normal subjects and carriers is often considerable, and the sensitivity of this type of test is only moderate.

The illustration of lens opacities was reproduced by kind permission of Professor P Harper, Institute of Medical Genetics for Wales, Cardiff.

SPECIAL ISSUES

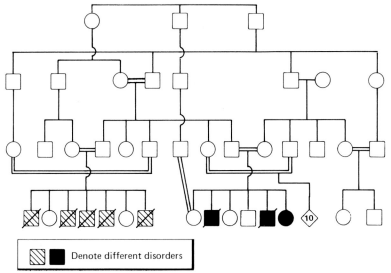

Denote different disorders

Autosomal recessive disorders in a family with complex consanguinity.

Various issues that arise during genetic counselling need special consideration and are briefly reviewed in this chapter. Consanguinity or disputed paternity affect the assessment of genetic risk, and families with genetic disorders need to know about adoption and other reproductive options. The study of twins has proved valuable in determining the genetic contribution to the aetiology of many disorders. In some genetic conditions population screening may be appropriate in the prevention or early detection of disease. The overall approach to genetic disorders raises various important ethical issues, which need to be faced by the family, the medical profession, and society.

Consanguinity

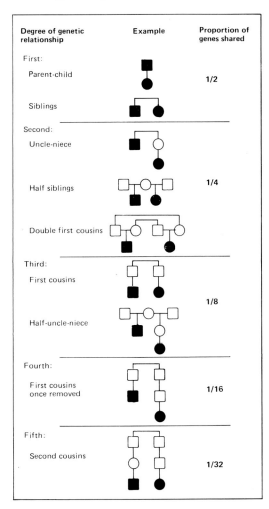

Consanguinity is a special problem in genetic counselling because of the increased risk of autosomal recessive disorders. Everyone probably carries at least one harmful autosomal recessive gene. In marriages between first cousins the chance of a child inheriting the same recessive gene from both parents that originated from one of the common grandparents and was transmitted through both sides of the family is one in 64. A different recessive gene may be similarly transmitted from the other common grandparent so that the risk of homozygosity for a recessive disorder in the child is one in 32. If two lethal genes are carried by each person the risk is one in 16.

Marriage between first cousins generally increases the risk of severe abnormality and mortality in offspring, by 3-5% compared with that in the general population. The increased risk associated with marriages between second cousins is around 1%.

Marriage between first and second degree relatives is almost universally illegal, although marriages between uncles and nieces occur in some Asian countries. Marriage between third degree relatives (between cousins or half uncles and nieces) is more common and permitted by law in many countries.

The offspring of incestuous relationships are at high risk of severe abnormality, mental retardation, and childhood death. Only about half of the children born to first degree relatives are normal, and this has important implications for termination of pregnancy or subsequent adoption.

Paternity

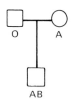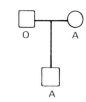

Non-paternity identified by blood group antigens.

Paternity not excluded by blood group antigens.

Clinical geneticists are sometimes asked to investigate disputed or uncertain paternity, particularly now that parentage can be accurately confirmed or excluded by DNA fingerprinting tests, which remove the uncertainty previously associated with analysis of blood groups. Testing of paternity, however, is not a clinical service, and disputed paternity remains a strictly legal issue.

Non-paternity may be discovered coincidentally during DNA testing of a family to investigate a mendelian disorder. Though this information must remain strictly confidential, it may substantially alter the risks to certain members of the family and is therefore of great importance in subsequent counselling.

Reproductive options

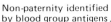

Pregnancy
- With or without prenatal diagnosis

Insemination by donor
- Existing child with autosomal recessive disorder
- Husband has autosomal dominant disorder
- Husband has chromosomal abnormality leading to infertility or recurrent spontaneous abortion

Ovum donation
- Wife has autosomal dominant or X linked disorder
- Wife has chromosomal abnormality leading to infertility or recurrent spontaneous abortion

Contraception
- Couples waiting for new medical developments

Sterilisation
- Couples whose family is complete

Various reproductive options are available to couples for whom pregnancy carries a high risk of abnormalities (box). The acceptability of any of these possibilities is a personal decision of the couple.

Adoption

A couple at risk of transmitting a genetic disorder may wish to consider adopting children as an alternative to pregnancy. The reduction in the availability of babies and young children for adoption should be realised, and, unfortunately, the presence of a genetic disorder in one of the couple may make this option more difficult to achieve. A rigorous assessment is made of prospective adoptive parents, and application takes at least a year. The chances of successful adoption are greater for couples able to accept older children or children with identified problems or handicaps.

A child placed for adoption may have a family history of a genetically determined disease, such as schizophrenia, and this may indeed be the reason for adoption. Some serious genetic disorders can be identified in infancy, others may not become apparent until adult life. Assessing the risk to the child before adoption is important, and adoptive parents should be given appropriate information about the risks and their implications. Generally, children with confirmed genetic disorders or those at risk should not be considered to be unsuitable for adoption as many adoptive parents elect to proceed with adoption after the possibilities for the child's future have been discussed.

Twins

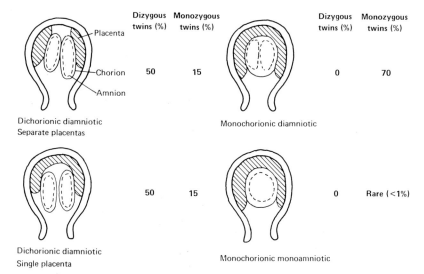

	Dizygous twins (%)	Monozygous twins (%)		Dizygous twins (%)	Monozygous twins (%)
Dichorionic diamniotic Separate placentas	50	15	Monochorionic diamniotic	0	70
Dichorionic diamniotic Single placenta	50	15	Monochorionic monoamniotic	0	Rare (<1%)

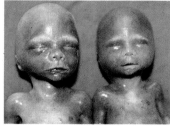

Twin fetuses discordant for Down's syndrome (affected twin on right).

Twins may be derived from a single egg (monozygous, identical) or two separate eggs (dizygous, fraternal). Examination of the placenta and membranes may help to distinguish between monozygous and dizygous twins but is not completely reliable. Monozygosity—resulting in twins of the same sex who look alike—can be confirmed by investigating inherited characteristics such as blood group markers or DNA polymorphisms (fingerprinting).

Dizygous twins may be familial and are more common in blacks than in white Europeans. Monozygous twins are seldom familial and have a fairly constant incidence of 0·4% of pregnancies. Monozygous twin pregnancies are associated with twice the risk of congenital malformation as singleton or dizygous twin pregnancies.

Twins share a common intrauterine environment, but though monozygous twins are genetically identical, dizygous twins are no more alike than any other pair of siblings. This provides the basis for studying twins to determine the genetic contribution in various disorders, by comparing the rates of concordance or discordance for a particular trait between pairs of monozygous and dizygous twins. The rate of concordance in monozygous twins is high for disorders in which genetic predisposition plays a major part in the aetiology of the disease. The phenotypic variability of genetic traits can be studied in monozygous twins, and the effect of a shared intrauterine environment may be studied in dizygous twins.

Screening for genetic disorders

Screening for carriers
Thalassaemia

Sickle cell disease

Tay-Sachs disease

Screening pregnancies at risk
Neural tube defect

Down's syndrome

Neonatal screening
Phenylketonuria

Hypothyroidism

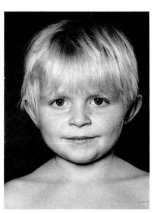

Child of normal intelligence
treated for phenylketonuria.

Screening programmes may be designed to diagnose genetic disorders or to identify couples at risk of transmitting genetic disorders to their children. Screening tests must be sufficiently sensitive to avoid false negative results and yet specific enough to avoid false positive results. To be employed on a large scale the tests must also be safe, simple, and fairly inexpensive. Screening programmes need to confer benefits to individual subjects as well as to society and to be successful stigmatisation must be avoided.

High risk subgroups of the population can be screened to identify carriers of recessive genes for a few disorders, notably, haemoglobinopathies and Tay-Sachs disease, and this allows prenatal diagnosis to be offered during pregnancy before the couple have an affected child. A screening programme for carriers of cystic fibrosis will be appropriate once a reliable test to detect carriers is available.

Screening during pregnancy for neural tube defect is offered by many obstetric centres. Estimation of maternal serum α fetoprotein concentration identifies over 90% of fetuses with anencephaly and around 80% of those with open neural tube defect. Screening for Down's syndrome is generally based on maternal age and does not identify all cases. A detection rate of 35% could be achieved if all women aged over 35 had amniocentesis during their pregnancy. The rate of detection can be improved by incorporating the results of measurements of serum α fetoprotein, unconjugated oestriol, and human chorionic gonadotrophin concentrations with maternal age to give a composite risk value, but this refinement is not currently available as a screening programme.

There are well established programmes for screening all neonates for phenylketonuria and hypothyroidism, and early diagnosis and treatment is successful in preventing mental retardation in the affected children. The value of including other metabolic disorders in a screening programme would depend on the incidence of the disorder and the prospect of altering the prognosis by its early detection. Possible candidates include galactosaemia, maple syrup urine disease, and congenital adrenal hyperplasia.

Ethical issues

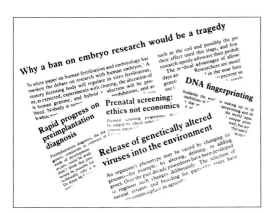

Many ethical controversies occur in clinical genetics. Predictive genetic testing, embryo research, and potential gene therapy are some that are currently debated. New technologies often generate concern over their potential application and safety. Widely publicised fears about the possible danger of genetic engineering accidents have proved unfounded, and recombinant DNA technology now plays an important part in investigating genetic disease.

In clinical practice the preservation of patient confidentiality may conflict with the need to disclose particular information to other family members. If a patient refuses to allow information about himself or herself to be disclosed the doctor may have to break confidentiality to inform immediate relatives of their own risk of developing or transmitting a disorder. Moral dilemmas also face many families with genetic disorders—for example, couples may have to make decisions about prenatal diagnosis and termination of pregnancy. Personal convictions about such issues vary widely, and it is important that couples should be allowed to make their own decisions with the help of non-directive medical information.

The illustration of the twin fetuses discordant for Down's syndrome was reproduced by kind permission of Dr Dian Donnai, St Mary's Hospital, Manchester.

CHROMOSOMAL DISORDERS I

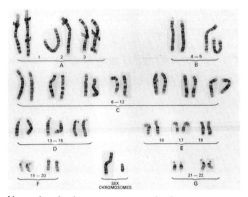

Normal male chromosome constitution.

The correct chromosome complement in humans was established in 1956, and the first chromosomal disorders (Down's, Turner's, and Klinefelter's syndromes) were defined in 1959. Since then refinements in techniques of preparing and examining samples have led to the description of hundreds of disorders that are due to chromosomal abnormalities.

Description of terms

Euploid	Chromosome numbers are multiples of the haploid set (2n)
Polyploid	Chromosome numbers are greater than diploid (3n, triploid)
Aneuploid	Chromosome numbers are not exact multiples of the haploid set (2n+1 trisomy; 2n−1 monosomy)
Mosaic	Presence of two different cell lines derived from one zygote (46XX/45X, Turner's mosaic)
Chimaera	Presence of two different cell lines derived from fusion of two zygotes (46XX/46XY, true hermaphrodite)

Human somatic cells contain 46 chromosomes organised into 22 autosomal pairs plus sex chromosomes. The basic haploid set (n=23) is present in the gametes. After fertilisation the zygote contains a diploid set of chromosomes (2n=46); one of each pair is maternal in origin, the other paternal.

During meiosis, which is the nuclear division giving rise to the gametes, recombination occurs between homologous parental chromosomes. The exchange of chromosomal material leads to the separation of genes originally located on the same chromosome, and gives rise to genetic variation within families.

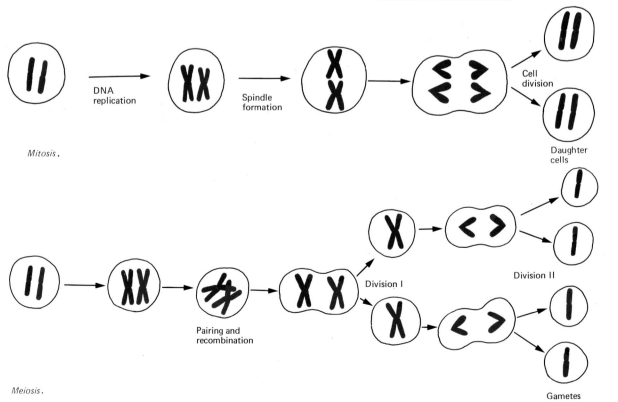

Mitosis.

Meiosis.

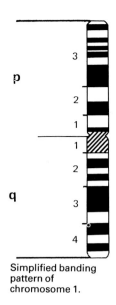

Simplified banding
pattern of
chromosome 1.

Each chromosome can be identified by light microscopy with staining techniques that give a characteristic pattern of alternating light and dark bands. During metaphase the two chromatids of each chromosome are joined at the centromere. The short arm of the chromosome is designated p and the long arm q. Each arm is subdivided numerically into a number of bands, according to the Paris convention, which permits precise localisation of a structural abnormality. High resolution cytogenetic techniques have permitted identification of small interstitial chromosome deletions in recognised disorders of previously unknown origin, such as Prader-Willi and Angelman's syndromes. Deletions too small to be detected by microscopy may be amenable to diagnosis by DNA techniques.

Types of chromosomal disorders

Type of disorder	Example		Outcome
Numerical			
Polyploid	Triploidy	69 chromosomes	Lethal
Aneuploid	Trisomy of chromosome 21		Down's syndrome
	Monosomy of X chromosome		Turner's syndrome
	47 chromosomes (XXY)		Klinefelter's syndrome
Structural			
Deletion	Terminal deletion 5p		Cri du chat syndrome
	Interstitial deletion 11p		Found in Wilms's tumour
Inversion	Pericentric inversion 9		Normal phenotype
Duplication	Isochromosome X (fusion of long arms with loss of short arms)		Infertility in females
Ring chromosome	Ring chromosome 18		Mental retardation syndrome
Fragile site	Fragile X		Mental retardation syndrome
Translocation	Reciprocal		Balanced translocations cause no abnormality. Unbalanced translocations cause spontaneous abortions or syndromes of multiple physical and mental handicaps
	Robertsonian		

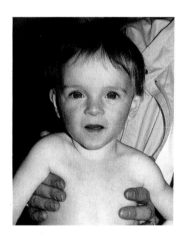

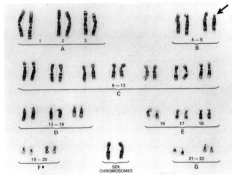

Cri du chat syndrome associated with deletion of short arm of chromosome 5.

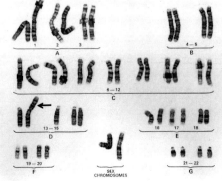

Balanced Robertsonian translocation affecting chromosomes 13 and 14.

Reporting of karyotypes

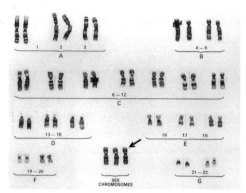

47XXX karyotype in triple X syndrome.

- Total number of chromosomes given first followed by constitution of sex chromosomes:

46XX   Normal female
47XXY Male with Klinefelter's syndrome
47XXX Female with triple X syndrome

- Additional or lost chromosomes are indicated by + or −:

47XY+21   Male with trisomy 21 (Down's syndrome)
46XX12p+ Additional unidentified material on short arm of chromosome 12

- All cell lines present are shown for mosaics:

46XX/47XX+21   Down's mosaic
46XX/47XXX/45X Turner's/triple X mosaic

- Structural rearrangements are described, identifying p and q arms and location of abnormality:

46XY del 11 (p13)   Deletion of short arm of chromosome 11 at band 13
46XX t (X;7) (p21;q23) Translocation between chromosome X and 7 with break points in respective chromosomes

Incidence of chromosomal abnormalities

Incidence of chromosomal abnormalities in spontaneous abortions and stillbirths

	%
Spontaneous abortions:	
All	50
Before 12 weeks	60
12-20 Weeks	20
Stillbirths	5

Types of chromosomal abnormalities in spontaneous abortions

	%
Trisomy	52
Monosomy X	18
Triploidy	17
Translocations	2-4

Chromosomal abnormalities are particularly common in spontaneous abortions. About 15-20% of all conceptions are estimated to be lost spontaneously, and about half of these are associated with a chromosomal abnormality. Most chromosomal abnormalities lead to spontaneous abortion, some inevitably so—for example, trisomy 16 is commonly found in aborted fetuses but never in liveborn infants.

Chromosomal abnormalities in newborn infants (per 1000)

All	6·5
Autosomal trisomy	1·7
Autosomal rearrangements	1·9
Other autosomal abnormality	0·4
Sex chromosomal	2·5

Common abnormalities

Autosomal
Trisomy 21—Down's
Trisomy 18—Edwards's   } syndrome
Trisomy 13—Patau's

Sex chromosomal
XO—Turner's
XXX—Triple X   } syndrome
XXY—Klinefelter's
XYY—XYY Male

In liveborn infants chromosomal abnormalities occur at about six per 1000 births. The incidence of abnormalities of autosomes and sex chromosomes is about the same. The effect on the child depends on the type of abnormality. Abnormalities do not occur in balanced rearrangements and are mild in disorders of the sex chromosomes. Unbalanced autosomal abnormalities cause disorders with multiple congenital malformations, almost invariably associated with mental retardation.

The illustrations of normal male, cri du chat, Robertsonian translocation 13;14, and triple X karyotypes were reproduced by kind permission of Dr Lorraine Gaunt, St Mary's Hospital, Manchester.

CHROMOSOMAL DISORDERS II

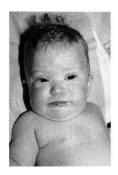

Child with developmental delay and deletion of chromosome 13.

Chromosomal abnormalities generally cause multiple congenital malformations and mental retardation. Children with more than one physical abnormality, particularly if retarded, should therefore undergo chromosomal analysis as part of their investigation. Chromosomal disorders are incurable but can be reliably detected by prenatal diagnostic techniques. Amniocentesis or chorionic villus sampling should be offered to women whose pregnancies are at increased risk—namely, women in their mid to late thirties, couples with an affected child, and couples in whom one partner carries a balanced translocation. Unfortunately, when there is no history of previous abnormality the risk in many affected pregnancies cannot be predicted before the child is born.

Autosomal abnormalities

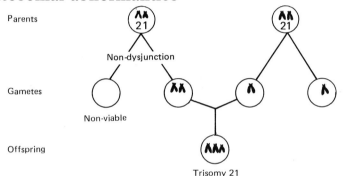

Non-dysjunction of chromosome 21 leading to Down's syndrome.

Trisomy 21 (Down's syndrome)

Down's syndrome is the commonest autosomal trisomy, the incidence in liveborn infants being one in 650, although more than half of conceptions with trisomy 21 do not survive to term. Affected children have a characteristic facial appearance, are mentally retarded, and may die young. They may have associated congenital heart disease and are at increased risk for recurrent infections, atlantoaxial instability, and acute leukaemia.

Most cases are due to non-dysjunction of chromosome 21 during meiosis in the formation of eggs or sperm. Although occurring at any age, non-dysjunction increases with maternal age. The risk of recurrence for a chromosomal abnormality in a liveborn infant after the birth of a child with trisomy 21 is about 1% (0·5% for trisomy 21 and 0·5% for other chromosomal abnormalities). For mothers aged 35 and over the total risk is around four times the risk related to age quoted in the table, half being for Down's syndrome and half for other chromosomal abnormalities.

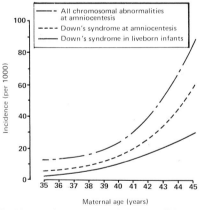

Incidence of chromosomal abnormalities and Down's syndrome by maternal age.

Risk for trisomy 21 in liveborn infants by maternal age

Maternal age at delivery	Risk
All ages	1 in 650
Age 30	1 in 900
Age 35	1 in 400
Age 36	1 in 300
Age 37	1 in 250
Age 38	1 in 200
Age 39	1 in 150
Age 40	1 in 100
Age 44	1 in 40

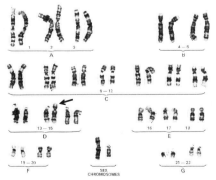

Down's syndrome due to Robertsonian translocation between chromosomes 14 and 21.

About 5% of cases of Down's syndrome are due to translocation, in which chromosome 21 is translocated on to chromosome 14 or, occasionally, chromosome 22. In less than half of these cases one of the parents has a balanced version of the same translocation. A healthy adult with a balanced translocation has 45 chromosomes, and the affected child has 46 chromosomes, the extra chromosome 21 being present in the translocation form.

The risk of Down's syndrome in the offspring is 10% when the balanced translocation is carried by the mother and 2·5% when carried by the father. If neither parent has a balanced translocation, an affected child represents a spontaneous, newly arising event, and the risk of recurrence is low (<1%).

Chromosomal disorders II

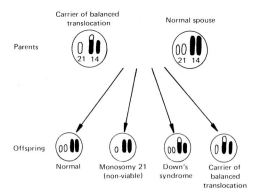

Parents — Carrier of balanced translocation — Normal spouse

Offspring — Normal — Monosomy 21 (non-viable) — Down's syndrome — Carrier of balanced translocation

Possible chromosome arrangements in offspring of a carrier of a balanced 14;21 translocation.

Occasionally, Down's syndrome is due to a 21;21 translocation. A parent with a balanced translocation would be unable to have normal children.

When a case of translocation occurs it is important to test other family members to identify all carriers of the translocation whose pregnancies would be at risk.

Couples concerned about a family history of Down's syndrome can have their chromosomes analysed from a sample of blood to exclude a balanced translocation if the karyotype of the affected person is not known. This usually avoids unnecessary amniocentesis during pregnancy.

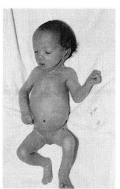

Trisomy 18—skull shape and facial features, short sternum, clenched hands, and rocker-bottom feet.

Trisomy 18 (Edwards's syndrome)

Trisomy 18 has an overall incidence of around 0·12 per 1000 live births. As with Down's syndrome most cases are due to non-dysjunction and the incidence increases with maternal age. Risk of recurrence is low, unless due to a parental translocation. Affected infants usually succumb within a few weeks or months but may occasionally survive several years. The main features include mental deficiency, growth deficiency, characteristic facial appearance, clenched hands, rocker bottom feet, and cardiac and renal abnormalities.

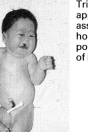

Trisomy 13—facial appearance associated with holoprosencephaly; postaxial polydactyly of hands and feet.

Trisomy 13 (Patau's syndrome)

The incidence of trisomy 13 is about 0·07 per 1000 live births, mainly due to non-dysfunction, with low risk of recurrence. Cases of translocation with higher risk of recurrence also occur. Most affected infants succumb within hours or weeks of birth. The main features include severe mental deficit; structural abnormalities of the brain, including microcephaly and holoprosencephaly (a developmental defect of the forebrain); cleft lip and palate; polydactyly; and ophthalmic, cardiac, and renal malformations.

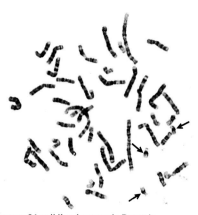

Trisomy 21 cell line in mosaic Down's syndrome. (Normal cell line also present.)

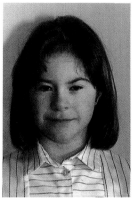

Girl with mosaic trisomy 21.

Mosaics

After fertilisation of a normal egg non-dysfunction may occur during a mitotic division in the developing embryo. This results in a fetus with two populations of cells. In Down's mosaicism one cell line has a normal constitution of 46 chromosomes and the other has a constitution of 47+21. The proportion of each cell line varies among different tissues. The proportion of trisomic cells present influences the phenotypic expression of the disorder, which is generally milder than in full trisomy.

In subjects with mosaic chromosomal abnormalities the abnormal cell line may not be present in peripheral lymphocytes, and skin biopsy and culturing of the cells is often required for diagnosis.

The clinical importance of a mosaic abnormality that is detected by amniocentesis can be difficult to interpret. Mosaicism of chromosome 20, for example, is not usually associated with fetal abnormality. Mosaicism for a marker (small unidentified) chromosome carries a much smaller risk of causing mental retardation if familial, and therefore the parents need to be investigated before advice can be given. Mosaicism detected in chorionic villus samples may reflect an abnormality confined to placental tissue that does not affect the fetus.

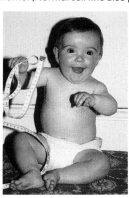

Normal 8 month old infant born after trisomy 20 mosaicism detected in amniotic cells.

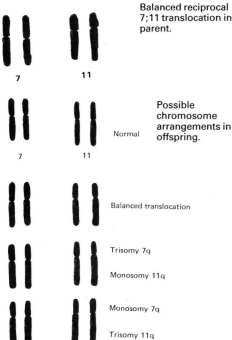

Balanced reciprocal 7;11 translocation in parent.

7   11

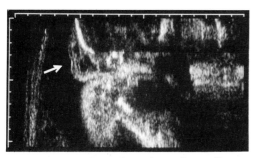

Normal

Possible chromosome arrangements in offspring.

7   11

Balanced translocation

Trisomy 7q

Monosomy 11q

Monosomy 7q

Trisomy 11q

Reciprocal translocations

Abnormalities resulting from an unbalanced translocation karyotype depend on the particular chromosome fragments that are present in monosomic or trisomic form. Sometimes spontaneous abortion is inevitable; at other times a child with multiple abnormalities may be born alive. The risk of an unbalanced karyotype occurring in offspring depends on the individual translocation.

Once a translocation has been identified it is important to investigate relatives of that person to identify carriers of the balanced translocation whose offspring would be at risk. Pregnancies can be monitored with chorionic villus sampling or amniocentesis.

Sex chromosomal abnormalities

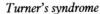

Cystic hygroma in Turner's syndrome detected by ultrasonography.

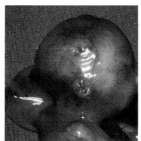

Fetus with Turner's syndrome.

Numerical abnormalities of the sex chromosomes are fairly common and cause less severe defects than autosomal abnormalities. They are often detected coincidentally at amniocentesis or during investigation for infertility, and risk of recurrence in families is low. When more than one additional sex chromosome is present mental retardation or physical abnormality is more likely.

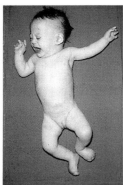

Lymphoedema of the feet as only manifestation of Turner's syndrome in newborn infant.

Turner's syndrome

Turner's syndrome results in early spontaneous loss of the fetus in over 95% of cases. Severely affected fetuses who survive to the second trimester can be detected by ultrasonography, which shows cystic hygroma, chylothorax, ascites, and hydrops.

The incidence of Turner's syndrome in liveborn female infants is 0·4 per 1000. Phenotypic abnormalities vary considerably but are usually mild. In some infants the only detectable abnormality is lymphoedema of the hands and feet. The most consistent features of the syndrome are short stature and infertility, but neck webbing, cubitus valgus, and aortic coarctation may also occur. Intelligence is usually within the normal range, but a few girls have educational problems. Growth can be stimulated with androgens or growth hormone, and oestrogen replacement treatment is necessary for pubertal development.

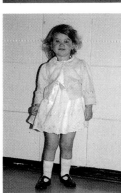

Normal appearance and development in 22 month girl with triple X syndrome.

Triple X syndrome

The triple X syndrome occurs with an incidence of 0·65 per 1000 liveborn female infants and is usually a coincidental finding. Apart from being taller than average, affected girls are physically normal. Educational problems are encountered more often in this group than in the other types of sex chromosomal abnormalities. Mean intelligence quotient is lower than in controls, about half of affected girls having delayed speech development and three quarters requiring some remedial teaching. Gonadal function is usually normal, but premature ovarian failure may occur.

Chromosomal disorders II

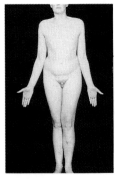

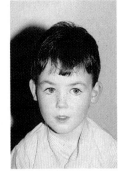

Tall stature, truncal obesity, and underdeveloped genitalia in Klinefelter's syndrome.

Normal facial appearance in mildly retarded boy with 48XYYY karyotype.

Klinefelter's syndrome

The XXY karyotype of Klinefelter's syndrome occurs with an incidence of 2·0 per 1000 liveborn males. The primary feature of the syndrome is hypogonadism, and affected males are usually tall. Pubertal development often progresses normally, but testosterone replacement treatment is sometimes required. Testicular size decreases after puberty, and affected males are infertile. Gynaecomastia may occur, and the risk of cancer of the breast is increased. Intelligence is generally within the normal range, but educational difficulties and behavioural problems are fairly common.

XYY syndrome

The XYY syndrome occurs in about 1·5 per 1000 liveborn male infants. Although more prevalent among inmates of high security institutions, the syndrome is less strongly associated with aggressive behaviour than previously thought, and many affected males remain undetected clinically. Mild mental retardation and behavioural problems can occur, and tall stature is usual.

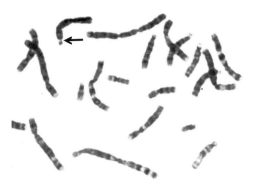

Fragile X chromosome.

Fragile X syndrome

The fragile X syndrome, first described in 1969 and delineated during the mid-1970s, is the most common single cause of severe mental retardation after Down's syndrome. Analysis of chromosomes with special culture techniques identifies a fragile site near the end of the long arm of the X chromosome in a proportion of cells in affected males and in female carriers.

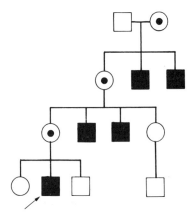

X linked recessive pedigree in fragile X syndrome.

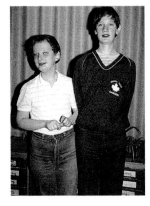

Mentally retarded brothers with fragile X syndrome.

The syndrome is inherited as an X linked disorder. Affected males usually have severe mental retardation (intelligence quotient 20-80, mean 50). Physical characteristics include macro-orchidism, prominent forehead, and large jaw and ears. The incidence in males is about 1·0 per 1000.

Mild to severe mental retardation also occurs in around 30% of heterozygous females. Not all female carriers show the chromosomal abnormality on testing, which makes counselling difficult in these families. Pregnancies at risk can currently be monitored with chorionic villus and fetal blood sampling for chromosome analysis, but in future DNA analysis will probably become the best method.

Illustrations reproduced by kind permission of colleagues at St Mary's Hospital, Manchester, were: Down's syndrome karyotype, Dr Lorraine Gaunt; fragile X karyotype, Mr M McKinley; cystic hygroma scan, Dr Sylvia Rimmer; trisomy 13, trisomy 18, Turner's syndrome fetus, and Klinefelter's syndrome, Dr Dian Donnai.

GENETICS OF COMMON DISORDERS

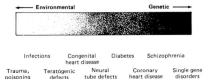

Relative contribution of environmental and genetic factors in some common disorders.

The genetic contribution to disease varies; some disorders are entirely environmental and others are wholly genetic. Many common disorders, however, have an appreciable genetic contribution but do not follow simple patterns of inheritance within a family. The terms multifactorial or polygenic inheritance have been used to describe the aetiology of these disorders. Normal traits inherited in this way include height and intelligence.

Multifactorial inheritance

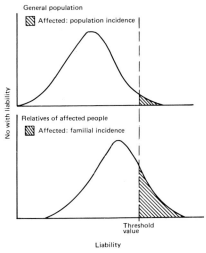

Hypothetical distribution of liability for a multifactorial disorder in general population and affected families.

The concept of multifactorial inheritance implies that a disease is caused by the interaction of several adverse genetic and environmental factors. The liability of a population to a particular disease follows a normal distribution curve, most people showing only moderate susceptibility and remaining unaffected. Only when a certain threshold of liability is exceeded is the disorder manifest. Relatives of an affected person will show a shift in liability, with a greater proportion of them being beyond the threshold. Familial clustering of a particular disorder may therefore occur.

Risk of recurrence

Factors increasing risk to relatives in multifactorial disorders

- High heritability of disorder
- Close relationship to proband
- Multiple affected family members
- Severe disease in proband
- Proband being of sex not usually affected

The risk of recurrence for a multifactorial disorder within a family is generally low and mainly affects first degree relatives. In many conditions family studies have reported the rate with which relatives of the proband have been affected. This allows empirical values for risk of recurrence to be calculated, which can be used in genetic counselling. A rational approach to preventing the disease is to modify known environmental triggers in genetically susceptible subjects. Vitamin supplementation in pregnancies at increased risk of neural tube defect and modifying diet and smoking habits in coronary heart disease are examples of effective intervention, but this approach is not currently possible for many disorders.

Heritability

Estimates of heritability

	Heritability (%)
Schizophrenia	85
Asthma	80
Cleft lip and palate	76
Coronary heart disease	65
Hypertension	62
Neural tube defect	60
Peptic ulcer	37

The genetic contribution to the aetiology of a disorder, or heritability, can be calculated from the disease incidence in the general population and that in relatives of an affected subject. Disorders with a greater genetic contribution have higher heritability and, hence, higher risks of recurrence.

HLA association and linkage

Diseases associated with histocompatibility antigens

Ankylosing spondylitis	B27
Autoimmune thyroid disease	B8, DR3
Chronic active hepatitis	B8, DR3
Coeliac disease	B8, DR3
Diabetes (juvenile)	{ B8, DR3 B15, DR4
Haemochromatosis	A3
Multiple sclerosis	DR2
Psoriasis	CW6
Reiter's disease	B27
Rheumatoid arthritis	DR4

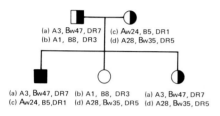

(a) A3, Bw47, DR7
(b) A1, B8, DR3

(c) Aw24, B5, DR1
(d) A28, Bw35, DR5

(a) A3, Bw47, DR7
(c) Aw24, B5,DR1

(b) A1, B8, DR3
(d) A28, Bw35, DR5

(a) A3, Bw47, DR7
(d) A28, Bw35, DR5

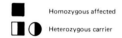

■ Homozygous affected

◧ ◖ Heterozygous carrier

Inheritance of congenital adrenal hyperplasia (21-hydroxylase deficiency) and HLA haplotypes (a) and (c).

Several important disorders occur more commonly than expected in subjects with particular HLA phenotypes, which implies that certain HLA determinants may affect disease susceptibility. Awareness of such associations may be helpful in counselling. For example, ankylosing spondylitis, which has an overall risk of recurrence of 4% in siblings, shows a strong association with HLA-B27, and 95% of affected people are positive for this antigen. The risk to their first degree relatives is increased to 9% for those who are also positive for HLA-B27 but reduced to less than 1% for those who are negative.

Genetic association, which may imply a causal relation, is different from genetic linkage, which occurs when two gene loci are physically close together on the chromosome. A disease gene, located near the HLA complex of genes on chromosome 6, will be linked to a particular HLA haplotype within a given affected family but will not necessarily be associated with the same HLA antigens in unrelated affected people. HLA typing can be used to predict disease by establishing the linked HLA haplotype within a given family.

Congenital adrenal hyperplasia due to 21-hydroxylase deficiency shows both linkage and association with histocompatibility antigens. The 21-hydroxylase gene lies within the HLA gene cluster and is therefore linked to the HLA haplotype. In addition, the salt losing form of 21-hydroxylase deficiency is associated with HLA-Bw47 antigen. This combination of linkage and association is known as linkage disequilibrium and results in certain alleles at neighbouring loci occurring together more often than would be expected by chance.

Diabetes

General distinction between insulin dependent and non-insulin dependent diabetes

	Insulin dependent diabetes	Non-insulin dependent diabetes
Clinical features	{ Thinness Ketosis Early onset	Obesity No ketosis Late onset
Treatment	Insulin	Diet or drugs
Concordance in monozygotic twins	50%	100%
Histocompatibility antigens	Associated	Not associated
Autoimmune disease	Associated	Not associated
Antibodies to insulin and Islet cells	Present	Absent

Factors indicating increased risk of insulin dependent diabetes

- HLA haplotypes shared with affected sibling
- DR3/DR4 antigens
- Insulin autoantibodies
- Islet cell antibodies
- Activated T lymphocytes

A genetic predisposition is well recognised in both type I insulin dependent diabetes and type II non-insulin dependent diabetes. Maturity onset diabetes of the young is a specific form of non-insulin dependent diabetes that follows autosomal dominant inheritance. Clinical diabetes or impaired glucose tolerance also occurs in several genetic syndromes—for example, haemochromatosis, growth hormone deficiency, and Wolfram syndrome (diabetes mellitus, optic atrophy, diabetes insipidus, and deafness). Only rarely is diabetes caused by the secretion of an abnormal insulin molecule.

Insulin dependent diabetes mellitus is heterogeneous, and the genetics of the disease is not clearly defined. Environmental factors, notably viral infections, are important, and only 50% of monozygous twins are concordant for the disease. An association with HLA-DR3 and HLA-DR4 phenotypes is well documented, with 95% of insulin dependent diabetics having one or both antigens compared with 50% of the normal population. Although the relative risk of developing diabetes for a person with HLA-DR3 or HLA-DR4 antigens is increased, most potentially susceptible people do not develop diabetes. The greatest risk is to subjects with two susceptibility antigens who have a family history of insulin dependent diabetes mellitus. Better definition of susceptible genotypes is becoming possible as subgroups of HLA-DR3 and HLA-DR4 serotypes are being identified by molecular analysis. An altered immune response controlled by genes closely linked to the class II HLA antigens may be responsible for susceptibility to the disease. Identifying people at risk with serological, immunological, or molecular markers will be important if presymptomatic preventive treatment becomes available.

Empirical risk for diabetes according to affected members of family

	Risk (%)
Insulin dependent diabetes:	
Sibling	3-10
One parent	3
Both parents	20
Monozygous twin	50
Non-insulin dependent diabetes:	
First degree relative	10-40
Monozygous twin	100
Maturity onset diabetes of the young:	
First degree relative	50

Non-insulin dependent diabetes mellitus shows a strong genetic predisposition, and concordance in monozygotic twins is almost 100%. The risk to siblings may approach 40% by the age of 80, but this high risk is for a disorder that is generally mild. The genetics of this type of diabetes are not understood, and genetically susceptible people cannot be identified with certainty, although certain alleles in the hypervariable region near the insulin gene detected by DNA analysis are found more commonly in non-insulin dependent diabetics than in the general population. Other factors, such as obesity, are also implicated in the aetiology.

Coronary heart disease

Types of hyperlipidaemia

	WHO type	Excess
Autosomal dominant:		
Familial hypercholesterolaemia	IIa, IIb	LDL
Familial combined hyperlipidaemia	IIa, IIb, IV	LDL, VLDL
Familial hypertriglyceridaemia	V, VI	VLDL, CM
Autosomal recessive:		
Apolipoprotein C II deficiency	I, V	CM, VLDL
Polygenic:		
Common hypercholesterolaemia	IIa	LDL

LDL=Low density lipoprotein; VLDL=very low density lipoprotein; CM=chylomicrons.

Environmental factors play a considerable part in coronary heart disease, but there is an underlying genetic susceptibility, and the risk to first degree relatives is increased to six times that of the general population. Lipoprotein abnormalities that increase the risk of heart disease may be secondary to dietary or other factors but often follow multifactorial inheritance.

Familial hypercholesterolaemia (type II hyperlipoproteinaemia) is dominantly inherited and may account for up to 10% of all early coronary heart disease. One in 500 of the general population are estimated to be heterozygous for the mutant gene. The risk of ischaemic heart disease increases with age in heterozygous subjects, who may also have xanthomas. Severe disease, often presenting in childhood, is seen in homozygous subjects.

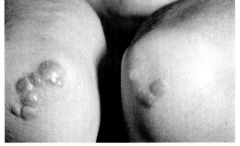
Xanthomas at elbows.

Familial aggregations of early coronary heart disease also occur in people without any detectable abnormality in lipid metabolism. Risks to relatives will be high and known environmental triggers should be avoided. Molecular genetic studies may lead to more precise identification of subjects at high risk by determining the major genes responsible.

Schizophrenia and affective psychoses

Overall incidence and empirical risk of recurrence (percentage) in schizophrenia and affective psychosis according to affected relative

	Schizophrenia	Affective psychosis
Incidence in general population	1	3
Sibling	9	13
One parent	13	15
Both parents	40	
Monozygous twin	40	70
Dizygous twin	10	15
Second degree relative	3	5

A strong familial tendency is found in both schizophrenia and affective disorders. The importance of genetic rather than environmental factors has been shown by reports of a high incidence of schizophrenia in children of affected parents and concordance in monozygotic twins, even when they are adopted and reared apart from their natural relatives. The same is true of manic depression. Empirical values for lifetime risk of recurrence are available for counselling, and the burden of the disorders needs to be taken into account. Both polygenic and single major gene models have been proposed to explain genetic susceptibility. A search for linked biochemical or molecular markers in large families with many affected members may be starting to identify major susceptibility genes.

Congenital malformations

Risk of recurrence in siblings for some common congenital malformations

	Risk (%)
Anencephaly or spina bifida	5*
Congenital heart disease	1-4
Cleft lip and palate	4
Cleft palate alone	2
Renal agenesis	3
Pyloric stenosis	2-10†
Congenital dislocated hip	1-11†
Club foot	3
Hypospadias	10
Cryptorchidism	10
Tracheo-oesophageal fistula	1
Exomphalos	<1

*Risk reduced by periconceptional supplementation with Pregnavite Forte F.
†Risk affected by sex of index case or sibling, or both.

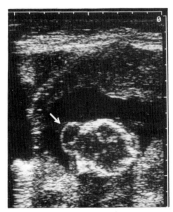

Occipital encephalocele detected by prenatal ultrasonography.

Mendelian, chromosomal, or teratogenic causes can be identified for many syndromes of multiple congenital abnormalities, and improved cytogenetic and DNA techniques will probably elucidate the cause in others. Some malformations are non-genetic, such as the amputations caused by early amniotic rupture. Many isolated congenital malformations, however, follow multifactorial inheritance, and the risk of recurrence depends on the specific malformation, its severity, and the number of affected people in the family. Decisions to have further children will be influenced by the fact that the risk of recurrence is generally low and that surgery for many isolated congenital malformations is successful. Prenatal ultrasonography may identify abnormalities requiring emergency neonatal surgery or severe malformations that have a poor prognosis, but it usually gives reassurance about the normality of a subsequent pregnancy.

Mental retardation

Risk of recurrence for severe non-specific mental retardation according to affected relative

	Risk
One sibling	1 in 35
One sibling with consanguineous parents	1 in 7
Two siblings	1 in 4
One parent	1 in 10
One sibling, one parent	1 in 5
Both parents	1 in 2
Male sibling, maternal uncle or male cousin	X linked

Intelligence is a polygenic trait, and mild mental retardation (intelligence quotient 50-70) represents the lower end of the normal distribution of intelligence. The intelligence quotient of offspring is likely to lie around the mid-parental mean. One or both parents of a mildly retarded child are often retarded themselves and have other retarded children. Intelligent parents with one mildly retarded child are unlikely to have another similarly affected child.

By contrast, the parents of a child with severe mental retardation (intelligence quotient <50) are usually of normal intelligence. A specific cause is more likely when the retardation is severe and may include chromosomal abnormalities and genetic disorders. The risk of recurrence depends on the diagnosis but in severe non-specific retardation is about 3% for siblings, increasing to 25% after the birth of two affected children.

The illustration of encephalocele was reproduced by kind permission of Dr Sylvia Rimmer, St Mary's Hospital, Manchester.

GENETICS OF CANCER

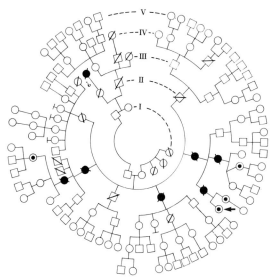

Autosomal dominant inheritance of ovarian adenocarcinoma.

Development of cancer is related to both environmental carcinogens and genetic predisposition. Though the risk of a common cancer occurring in relatives of an affected person is generally low, familial aggregations that cannot be explained by environmental factors alone exist in some neoplasms, such as breast and ovarian cancers and melanomas. In occasional families a predisposition to a combination of common cancers is inherited as an incompletely penetrant autosomal dominant trait. Several mendelian syndromes are also associated with a high risk of malignancy, although these are generally rare disorders. Chromosomal rearrangements may be markers for or the cause of certain neoplasias, and various oncogenes may be implicated. There is evidence that two mutational events are required for the development of some malignancies, one of which is inherited in familial cancers.

● Affected females
◉ Females at 50% risk having undergone prophylactic oophorectomy

Cancer family syndromes

Types of tumour in cancer family syndromes

Type 1		Type II	
Endometrium	Stomach	Breast	Lymphoma
Ovary	Pancreas	Sarcoma	Adrenal
Breast	Skin	Embryonal	Thyroid
Prostate	Melanoma	Brain	Bladder
Colon		Leukaemia	

Families can be identified in which many relatives develop malignancies, although the tumours may be of different types. One such instance is hereditary adenocarcinomatosis; another includes a predisposition to breast cancer, sarcomas, and embryonal tumours. The tumours develop earlier than usual, they may be multifocal, and more than one type of primary tumour may occur in the same person. The predisposition to cancer in these rare families behaves as an autosomal dominant trait with about 60% penetrance so that over 25% of descendants of the proband develop cancers. Identification of the families or their members at risk is not currently possible.

Mendelian cancer syndromes

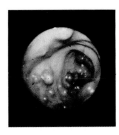

Colonic polyps in familial adenomatous polyposis.

Multiple polyposis syndromes

Polyposis coli follows autosomal dominant inheritance and carries a high risk of malignancy necessitating prophylactic colectomy. In familial adenomatous polyposis the intestinal polyps are the only feature of the disorder, but in Gardner's syndrome extracolonic manifestations including osteomas, epidermoid cysts, and various other tumours occur; the distinction between these two syndromes is unclear. Family members at risk should be screened with regular colonoscopy. Early identification of gene carriers may be possible by detecting congenital hypertrophy of the retinal pigment epithelium. The use of linked DNA markers on chromosome 5 also helps in detecting gene carriers and may avoid repeated colonoscopy in family members at low risk.

In Peutz-Jeghers syndrome hamartomatous gastrointestinal polyps, which may bleed or cause intussusception, are associated with pigmentation of the buccal mucosa and lips. The polyps are usually benign, but malignant degeneration occurs in about 5% of cases, mainly in gastric and duodenal polyps. Ovarian, breast, and endometrial tumours also occur in this dominant syndrome.

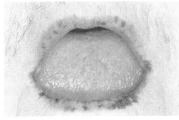

Pigmentation of lips in Peutz-Jeghers syndrome.

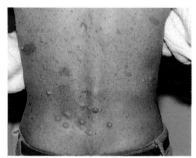

Peripheral neurofibromatosis.

Neurofibromatosis

Neurofibromatosis is the commonest disorder that is inherited as an autosomal dominant trait, with an incidence of one in 3000. The diagnostic criteria for peripheral neurofibromatosis (von Recklinghausen's disease) include the presence of café au lait patches and cutaneous neurofibromas. Benign optic gliomas and spinal neurofibromas may occur, and early detection facilitates their surgical removal. Malignant tumours, mainly neurofibrosarcomas or embryonal tumours, occur in about 5% of affected people. Central neurofibromatosis is also dominantly inherited, its main feature being bilateral acoustic neuromas. The genes for peripheral and central neurofibromatosis have been located on chromosomes 17 and 22, respectively.

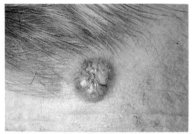

Heavily calcified intracranial hamartoma in tuberous sclerosis.

Tuberous sclerosis

Tuberous sclerosis is an autosomal dominant disorder, very variable in its manifestation, that can cause epilepsy and severe retardation in affected children. Hamartomas of the brain, heart, kidney, retina, and skin may also occur, and their presence indicates the carrier state in otherwise healthy family members. Sarcomatous malignant change is possible but uncommon. Linkage has been shown with chromosome 9 markers in some families.

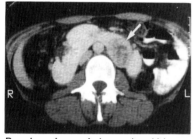

Basal cell carcinoma.

Naevoid basal cell carcinoma syndrome

The cardinal features of the naevoid basal cell carcinoma syndrome, an autosomal dominant disorder delineated by Gorlin, are basal cell carcinomas, jaw cysts, and various skeletal abnormalities, including bifid ribs. Other features are macrocephaly, tall stature, palmar pits, calcification of the falx cerebri, ovarian fibromas, and other tumours. The skin tumours are usually bilateral and symmetrical, appearing over the face, neck, trunk, and arms during childhood or adolescence. Malignant change may occur, especially after the second decade, and removal of the tumours is therefore indicated.

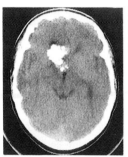

Renal carcinoma in horseshoe kidney on computed tomography in von Hippel-Lindau disease.

von Hippel-Lindau disease

In von Hippel-Lindau disease haemangioblastomas develop throughout the brain and spinal cord, characteristically affecting the cerebellum and retina. Renal, hepatic, and pancreatic cysts also occur, and clear cell carcinoma of the kidney may develop; less common are phaeochromocytomas. The syndrome follows autosomal dominant inheritance, and yearly screening is recommended for affected family members or those at risk to permit early treatment of problems as they arise. Location of the gene on chromosome 3 will permit prediction of genetic state by DNA analysis.

Multiple endocrine neoplasia syndromes

Three main types of the multiple endocrine neoplasia syndrome exist and all follow autosomal dominant inheritance with reduced penetrance. Many affected people have involvement of more than one gland, and first degree relatives in affected families should be periodically screened to detect presymptomatic tumours. Abnormal calcitonin secretion in the type IIa syndrome, for example, can be detected by calcium or pentagastrin provocation tests, permitting curative thyroidectomy before the tumour cells extend beyond the thyroid capsule. Linkage between the type IIa syndrome and DNA markers on chromosome 10 has been shown and provides an additional method of predicting gene carriers.

Main types of multiple endocrine neoplasia

I	IIa	IIb
Parathyroid	Medullary thyroid	Medullary thyroid
Pancreatic islet cell	Phaeochromocytoma	Phaeochromocytoma
Pituitary	Parathyroid	Mucosal neuromas
Adrenal cortex		
Thyroid		

Inherited childhood tumours

Percentage risk of retinoblastoma in child according to affected relative

	Retinoblastoma
Bilateral tumours:	
Parent	40
Sibling	8
Unilateral tumour:	
Parent and another relative	40
Parent	6
Two siblings	40
One sibling	2

Two stages of tumour generation

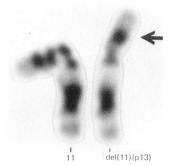

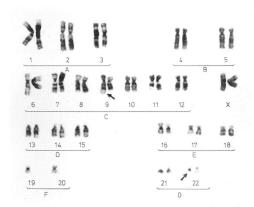

Deletion of chromosome 11 at band 11p13 in patient with Wilms's tumour.

Retinoblastoma

Most bilateral and about 15% of unilateral tumours seem to be hereditary. Inheritance follows an autosomal dominant pattern with incomplete penetrance; only about 80% of children with the abnormal gene develop retinoblastomas. Tumours may occasionally regress spontaneously leaving retinal scars, and parents of an affected child should be examined carefully. A deletion of chromosome 13, which has been found in some affected children who may have additional congenital abnormalities, has localised the retinoblastoma gene to chromosome 13q14. The esterase D locus is closely linked to the retinoblastoma locus and is a marker for identifying gene carriers in affected families as are recently identified DNA probes. Molecular studies indicate that two events are involved in the development of the tumour. In bilateral tumours the first mutation is inherited and the second is a somatic event. In unilateral tumours both events may represent new somatic mutations. The retinoblastoma gene is therefore acting recessively as mutant alleles at 13q14 on both chromosomes are needed for tumours to develop.

Second malignancies occur in up to 15% of survivors, more commonly in bilateral and familial cases. In addition to tumours of the head and neck caused by local irradiation treatment, other associated malignancies include sarcomas (particularly of the femur), pinealomas, and carcinomas of the bladder.

Wilms's tumour

Wilms's tumours are usually unilateral but may occasionally be bilateral. Recurrence within families is reported but is not very common. Inheritance seems to be autosomal dominant with reduced penetrance in these families. Aniridia occurs in 1% of patients with Wilms's tumour, and identification of an interstitial deletion of chromosome 11 in these patients has located a susceptibility gene to chromosome 11p13. As with retinoblastoma the tumours are homozygous for the deletion, indicating that two events are needed for tumours to develop. Hemihypertrophy occurs in about 3% of patients, and Wilms's tumour has also been reported in other disorders with growth disturbance such as neurofibromatosis and Beckwith-Wiedemann, Klippel-Trenaunay-Weber, and Sotos's syndromes. Various second primary malignancies may occur but are uncommon.

Chromosomal abnormalities in malignancy

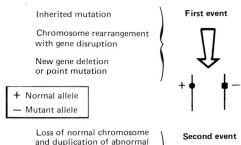

9;22 Translocation in chronic myeloid leukaemia. (One chromosome 19 and one chromosome 20 have also been lost from cell line.)

Structural chromosomal abnormalities are well documented in leukaemias and lymphomas and may be prognostic indicators. They are also evident in solid tumours—for example, an interstitial deletion of chromosome 3 occurs in small cell carcinoma of the lung. In addition, chromosome instability is seen in some autosomal recessive disorders that predispose to malignancy, such as ataxia telangiectasia, Fanconi's anaemia, xeroderma pigmentosum, and Bloom syndrome.

Philadelphia chromosome

The Philadelphia chromosome, found in blood and bone marrow cells, is a deleted chromosome 22 in which the long arm has been translocated on to the long arm of chromosome 9 and is designated t(9;22) (q34;q11). The translocation occurs in 90% of patients with chronic myeloid leukaemia, and its absence generally indicates a worse prognosis. The Philadelphia chromosome is also found in 10-15% of acute lymphocytic leukaemias, when its presence indicates a poor prognosis.

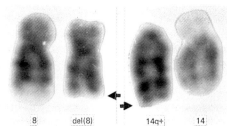

8;14 Translocation in Burkitt's lymphoma.

Burkitt's lymphoma

Burkitt's lymphoma is common in children in parts of tropical Africa. Infection with Epstein-Barr (EB) virus and chronic antigenic stimulation with malaria both play a part in the pathogenesis of the tumour. Most lymphoma cells carry an 8;14 translocation or occasionally a 2;8 or 8;22 translocation. The break points involve the cellular oncogene c-myc on chromosome 8 at 8q24, and the immunoglobulin heavy chain gene on chromosome 14 and $\varkappa$ and λ light chain genes on chromosomes 2 and 22 respectively. Altered activity of the oncogene when translocated into regions of immunoglobulin genes that are normally undergoing considerable recombination and mutation probably plays an important part in the development of the tumour.

Oncogenes

Some oncogene associations in chromosomal translocations in leukaemia

Disorder	Cytogenetic abnormality	Cellular oncogene and location	
Burkitt's lymphoma	t(8;14)(q24; q32) t(2;8)(p12;q24) t(8;22) (q24;q11)	c-myc	8q24
Chronic myeloid leukaemia	t(9;22)(q34;q11)	c-abl	9q34
Acute lymphocytic leukaemia	t(4;11)(q21;q23)	c-raf-2p c-ets 1	Chromosome 4 11q 23-24
Acute myeloid leukaemia	t(8;21)(q22;q22)	c-mos	8q22
Acute myeloid leukaemia (promyelocytic)	t(15;17)(q22;q11)	c-erb-A1	17q 11-21

Various oncogenes are implicated in the development of malignancy. Viral oncogenes (v-onc) are carried by RNA viruses (retroviruses) that can incorporate a DNA copy of their genomic RNA into host DNA. These viruses can transform host cells and were first recognised by their ability to cause neoplasms in animals.

Sequences homologous to those of the viral oncogenes in the human genome are called cellular oncogenes (c-onc). These oncogenes are important in normal growth and development of cells, but their mutation, amplification, or activation at inappropriate times may be involved in the initiation of neoplasia. Proteins encoded by oncogenes probably act within a cascade involving growth factors and may function as cell surface receptors or intracellular messengers or through production of protein kinases or nuclear proteins that bind to DNA.

Evidence exists for the role of cellular oncogenes in certain human cancers, notably c-myc in the translocation associated with Burkitt's lymphoma, c-abl in that of the Philadelphia chromosome, and N-myc amplification in neuroblastoma. Expression of oncogene products may become important in typing and staging tumours, contributing to definition of the prognosis and to treatment.

Illustrations reproduced by kind permission were: the ovarian adenocarcinoma pedigree, Drs Dian Donnai and D Warrell, St Mary's Hospital, Manchester; familial adenomatous polyposis from the *Slide Atlas of Gastroenterology*. Gower Medical Publishing, 1985 and Dr C Williams, St Mark's Hospital, London; the computed tomograms of tuberous sclerosis, Mr P Richardson, Manchester Royal Infirmary and University of Manchester, and renal carcinoma, Dr Judith Adams, University of Manchester Medical School; and the chromosome 11 deletion and 9;22 and 8;14 translocations, Dr Christine Harrison, Christie Hospital, Manchester.

DYSMORPHOLOGY AND TERATOGENESIS

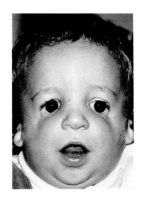

Treacher Collins syndrome: abnormal first branchial arch development giving rise to malar and mandibular hypoplasia with external ear malformations.

Dysmorphology is the study of malformations arising from abnormal embryogenesis. Recognition of patterns of multiple congenital malformations may allow inferences to be made about the timing, mechanism, and aetiology of structural defects. Animal research is providing information about cellular interactions, migration, and differentiation processes and gives insight into the possible mechanisms underlying human malformations. Diagnosing multiple congenital abnormalities in children can be difficult but is important to give correct advice about management, prognosis, and risk of recurrence.

Definition of terms

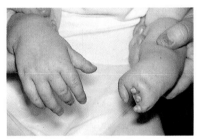

Unilateral terminal transverse defect of the hand occurring as an isolated malformation.

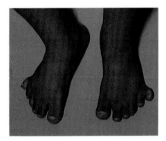

Postaxial polydactyly of the feet in Laurence-Moon-Biedl syndrome (obesity, mental retardation, polydactyly, retinitis pigmentosa, and genital hypoplasia).

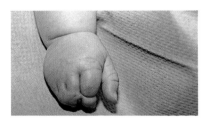

Constriction ring with amputation and fusion of digits caused by amniotic bands.

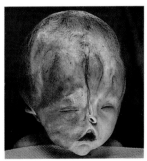

Severe disruption of the face caused by amniotic bands.

Malformation

A malformation is a primary structural defect occurring during development of an organ or tissue. An isolated malformation, such as cleft lip and palate, congenital heart disease, or pyloric stenosis, can occur in an otherwise normal child. Most single malformations are inherited as polygenic traits with a fairly low risk of recurrence, and corrective surgery is often successful. Multiple malformation syndromes comprise defects in two or more systems and are often associated with mental retardation. The risk of recurrence is determined by the aetiology, which may be chromosomal, teratogenic, due to a single gene, or unknown.

Disruption

A disruption defect implies that there is destruction of a part of a fetus that had initially developed normally. Amniotic band disruption after early rupture of the amnion is a well recognised entity, causing constriction bands and amputations of digits and limbs and sometimes more extensive disruptions causing, for example, facial clefts and central nervous system defects. As the fetus is genetically normal and the defects are caused by an extrinsic abnormality the risk of recurrence is small. Interruption of the blood supply to a developing part from other causes will also cause disruption owing to infarction with consequent atresia. The prognosis depends solely on the severity of the physical defect.

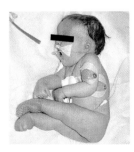

Deformation of legs in newborn infant with hypotonia due to congenital myotonic dystrophy.

Deformation

Deformations are due to abnormal intrauterine moulding and give rise to deformity of structurally normal parts. Deformations usually involve the musculoskeletal system and may occur in fetuses with congenital neuromuscular problems such as spinal muscular atrophy and congenital myotonic dystrophy. Paralysis in spina bifida gives rise to positional deformities of the legs and feet. In these disorders the prognosis is often poor and the risk of recurrence may be high.

Dysmorphology and teratogenesis

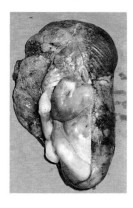
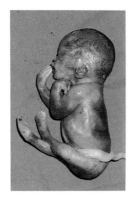

Fetal constraint and deformation due to oligohydramnios in Potter's syndrome (renal agenesis).

Oligohydramnios causes fetal deformation and is well recognised in fetal renal agenesis (Potter's syndrome). The absence of urine production by the fetus results in severe oligohydramnios, which in turn causes fetal deformation and pulmonary hypoplasia. Oligohydramnios caused by chronic leakage of liquor has a similar effect.

A normal fetus may be constrained by uterine abnormalities, breech presentation, or multiple pregnancy. The prognosis is generally excellent, and the risk of recurrence is low except in cases of structural uterine abnormality.

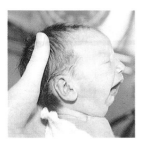

Pierre Robin sequence: mandibular hypoplasia causing cleft palate and respiratory obstruction.

Sequence

The term sequence implies that a series of events occur after a single initiating abnormality, which may be a malformation, a deformation, or a disruption. The features of Potter's syndrome can be classed as a malformation sequence in which the initial abnormality is renal agenesis, which gives rise to secondary deformation and pulmonary hypoplasia. Other examples are the holoprosencephaly sequence and the sirenomelia sequence. In holoprosencephaly the primary developmental defect is in the forebrain, leading to microcephaly, absent olfactory and optic nerves, and midline defects in facial development, including hypotelorism or cyclopia, midline cleft lip, and abnormal development of the nose. In sirenomelia the primary defect affects the caudal axis of the fetus, from which the lower limbs, bladder, genitalia, kidneys, hindgut, and sacrum develop. Abnormalities of all these structures occur in the sirenomelia sequence.

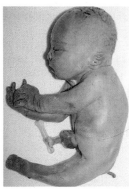

Sirenomelia sequence: fused legs, tail like appendage, absent genitalia, imperforate anus, exomphalos, and renal agenesis.

Associations

Certain malformations occur together more often than expected by chance alone; these are termed associations. The names given to recognised malformation associations are often acronyms of the component abnormalities. Hence the *Vater* association consists of *v*ertebral anomalies, *a*nal atresia, *t*racheo-oesophageal fistula, and *r*adial defects. The acronym *vacterl* has been suggested to encompass the additional *c*ardiac, *r*enal, and *l*imb defects of this association.

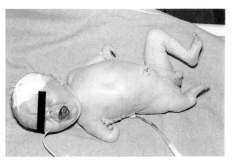

Vater association.

Murcs association is the name given to the non-random occurrence of *Mü*llerian duct aplasia, *r*enal aplasia, and *c*ervicothoracic *s*omite dysplasia. In the *Charge* association the related abnormalities include *c*olobomas of the eye, *h*eart defects, *a*tresia choanae, mental *r*etardation, *g*rowth retardation, and *e*ar anomalies.

Identification of syndromes

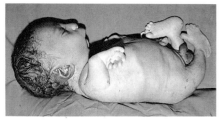

Robert's syndrome: autosomal recessive "pseudothalidomide" syndrome with hypomelia, mid-facial defect, and severe growth deficiency.

Patterns of multiple malformations that occur together constitute syndromes. Recognition of syndromes is important to answer the questions that parents of all babies with congenital malformations ask—namely,

What is it?

Why did it happen?

What does it mean for the child's future?

Will it happen again?

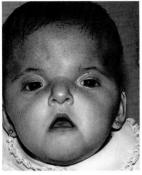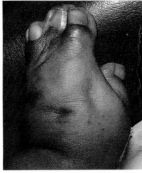

Apert's syndrome: autosomal dominant craniosynostosis with fused digits.

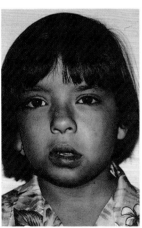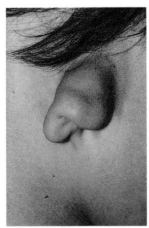

Smith-Lemli-Opitz syndrome: autosomal recessive syndrome with ptosis, anteverted nares, syndactyly of second and third toes, hypospadias, and mental retardation.

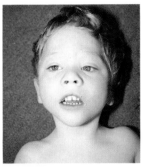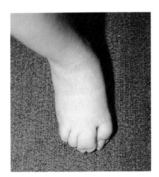

Goldenhar's syndrome (hemifacial microsomia): usually sporadic syndrome with asymmetrical malar, maxillary, and mandibular hypoplasia and microtia.

Stillbirths

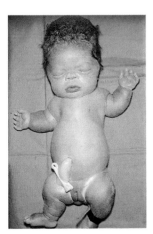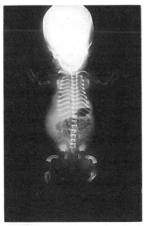

Thanatophoric dwarfism: usually sporadic lethal bone dysplasia.

Parents experience feelings of grief and guilt after the birth of an abnormal child, and time spent discussing what is known about the aetiology of the abnormalities may help to alleviate some of their fears. They also need an explanation of what to expect in terms of treatment, anticipated complications, and long term outlook. Accurate assessment of the risk of recurrence cannot be made without a diagnosis, and the availability of prenatal diagnosis in subsequent pregnancies will depend on whether there is an associated chromosomal abnormality or a structural defect amenable to detection by ultrasonography.

The assessment of infants and children with malformations requires careful taking of a history and a physical examination. Abnormalities during the pregnancy, including possible exposure to teratogens, should be recorded, as well as the occurrence of any perinatal problems. Parental age and family history may provide clues about the aetiology. Examination of the child should include detailed documentation of the abnormalities present with accurate clinical measurements and photographic records whenever possible, and the investigations required may include chromosomal analysis and biochemical or radiological studies.

A chromosomal or mendelian aetiology has been identified for many multiple congenital malformation syndromes. When the aetiology of a recognised multiple malformation syndrome is not known empirical figures for the risk of recurrence derived from family studies can be used, and these are usually fairly low. Consanguineous marriages may give rise to autosomal recessive syndromes unique to a particular family: when more than one child is affected counselling the couple using the one in four risk of recurrence associated with autosomal recessive inheritance is appropriate.

Numerous malformation syndromes have been identified, and many are extremely rare. Published case reports and specialised texts may have to be reviewed before diagnosis. Computer programs are now available to assist in differential diagnosis, but despite this syndromes in a proportion of children will inevitably remain undiagnosed.

Detailed examination and investigation of malformed stillbirths and fetuses is essential if parents are to be accurately counselled about the cause of the problem, the risk of recurrence, and the availability of prenatal tests in future pregnancies. As with liveborn infants careful documentation of the abnormalities is required with detailed photographic records. Cardiac blood samples and skin biopsy specimens should be taken for chromosome analysis and bacteriological and virological investigations performed. Other investigations, including full skeletal x ray examination and tissue sampling for biochemical studies and DNA extraction, may be necessary. Necropsy will determine the presence of associated internal abnormalities, which may permit diagnosis.

Environmental teratogens

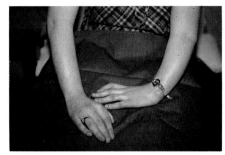

Limb malformation due to intrauterine exposure to thalidomide.

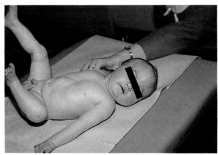

Hypospadias, congenital heart disease, prominent metopic suture (trigonocephaly), and psychomotor retardation in the fetal valproate syndrome.

Examples of teratogens

- *Drugs*
  Alcohol
  Anticonvulsants
  　Phenytoin
  　Sodium valproate
  Anticoagulants
  　Warfarin
  Antibiotics
  　Streptomycin
  Treatment for acne
  　Tetracycline
  　Isotretinoin
  Antimalarials
  　Chloroquine
  　Pyrimethamine
  Anticancer drugs
  Androgens

- *Environmental chemicals*
  Organic $\begin{cases} \text{mercurials} \\ \text{solvents} \end{cases}$

- *Radiation*

- *Maternal disorders*
  Epilepsy
  Diabetes
  Phenylketonuria
  Hyperpyrexia
  Iodine deficiency

- *Intrauterine infection*
  Rubella
  Cytomegalovirus
  Toxoplasmosis
  Herpes simplex
  Varicella-zoster
  Syphilis

Drugs

Identification of drugs that cause fetal malformations is important as they constitute a potentially preventable cause of abnormality. Although fairly few drugs are proved teratogens in humans, and some drugs are known to be safe, the accepted policy is to avoid all drugs if possible during pregnancy. Thalidomide has been the most dramatic teratogen identified, and an estimated 10 000 babies world wide were damaged by this drug in the early 1960s before its withdrawal.

Alcohol is currently the most common teratogen, and studies suggest that between one in 300 and one in a 1000 infants are affected. Children with the fetal alcohol syndrome exhibit prenatal and postnatal growth deficiency, mental retardation, microcephaly, and characteristic facies with short palpebral fissures, a smooth philtrum, and a thin upper lip. In addition, they have tremulousness owing to withdrawal in the neonatal period.

Treatment of epilepsy during pregnancy presents particular problems as both phenytoin and sodium valproate are teratogenic and cause recognisable syndromes associated with mental retardation in a proportion of exposed pregnancies. Anticonvulsant treatment may be needed during pregnancy to avoid the risk of grand mal seizures, and it is not always possible to change to carbamazepine, which is currently thought to be the most suitable drug. Regardless of treatment, maternal epilepsy has been suggested to increase the risk of congenital abnormality in the offspring.

Maternal disorders

Several maternal disorders have been identified in which the risk of fetal malformations is increased including phenylketonuria and diabetes. In phenylketonuria the children of an affected woman will be healthy heterozygotes in relation to the abnormal gene, but if the mother is not returned to a carefully monitored diet before pregnancy the high maternal serum concentration of phenylalanine causes microcephaly in the developing fetus. The risk of congenital malformations in the pregnancies of diabetic women is two to three times higher than that in the general population but may be lowered by good diabetic control before conception and during the early part of pregnancy.

Intrauterine infection

Various intrauterine infections are known to cause congenital malformations in the fetus. Maternal infection early in gestation may cause structural abnormalities of the central nervous system, resulting in neurological abnormalities, visual impairment, and deafness, in addition to other malformations, such as congenital heart disease. When maternal infection occurs in late pregnancy the risk that the infective agent will cross the placenta is higher, and the newborn infant may present with signs of active infection, which include hepatitis, thrombocytopenia, haemolytic anaemia, and pneumonitis.

Rubella embryopathy is well recognised, and the aim of vaccination programmes against rubella virus during childhood is at reducing the number of non-immune girls reaching childbearing age. The presence of rubella specific IgM in fetal or neonatal blood samples identifies babies infected in utero. Cytomegalovirus is a common infection, and 5-6% of pregnant women may become infected. Only 3% of newborn infants, however, have evidence of cytomegalovirus infection, and no more than 5% of these develop subsequent problems. Natural infection with cytomegalovirus does not always confer immunity, and occasionally more than one sibling is affected by intrauterine infection. Unlike the case with rubella, vaccines against cytomegalovirus or toxoplasma are not available, and although active maternal toxoplasmosis can be treated with drugs such as pyrimethamine, this carries the risk of teratogenesis.

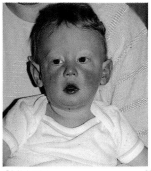

Child with
hepatosplenomegaly, delayed
development, and deafness
due to intrauterine
cytomegalovirus infection.

Herpes simplex infection in the newborn infant is generally acquired at the time of birth, but infection early in pregnancy is probably associated with an increased risk of abortion, late fetal death, prematurity, and structural abnormalities of the central nervous system. Maternal varicella infection may also affect the fetus, causing abnormalities of the central nervous system and cutaneous scars. The risk of a fetus being affected by varicella infection is not known but is probably less than 10%, with a critical period during the third and fourth months of pregnancy. Affected infants seem to have a high perinatal mortality rate.

The illustrations of disruption of the face caused by amniotic bands, congenital myotonic dystrophy, Pierre Robin sequence, sirenomelia sequence, Smith-Lemli-Opitz syndrome, thalidomide malformation, and the valproate syndrome were reproduced by kind permission of Dr Dian Donnai, St Mary's Hospital, Manchester. The illustrations of Potter's syndrome, the Vater association, and thanatophoric dwarfism were reproduced by kind permission of the University of Manchester and Dr Dian Donnai. The illustrations of Treacher Collins syndrome and Goldenhar's syndrome were reproduced from *Dental Update* by permission of Update-Siebert Publications.

PRENATAL DIAGNOSIS

Techniques for prenatal diagnosis

- Ultrasonography   —safe
  —performed in second trimester
- Amniocentesis   —procedure risk 0·5%
  —performed in second trimester
  —widely available
- Chorionic villus sampling   —procedure risk 2%
  —performed in first trimester
  —specialised technique
- Fetoscopy   —procedure risk 3%
  —performed in second trimester
  —very specialised technique
- Embryo biopsy   —future technique

Prenatal diagnosis is important in detecting and preventing genetic disease. Two main advances in recent years have been the development of chorionic villus sampling procedures in the first trimester and the application of recombinant DNA techniques to the diagnosis of many mendelian disorders. Various prenatal procedures are available, generally being performed between eight and 20 weeks' gestation. The timing, safety, and accuracy of prenatal tests are important factors that must be considered. Having prenatal tests and waiting for results is stressful for couples, and they must be supported during this time and given the results as soon as possible. Many couples who face a high risk of a serious genetic disorder in their children will consider embarking on a pregnancy only if reliable prenatal diagnosis is available. Prenatal testing may also be appropriate for couples in whom the pregnancies are at fairly low risk, often allowing a pregnancy to continue with less anxiety.

Indications for prenatal diagnosis

General criteria for prenatal diagnosis

- High genetic risk
- Severe disorder
- Treatment not available
- Reliable prenatal test
- Termination of pregnancy acceptable

Prenatal diagnosis occasionally allows prenatal treatment to be instituted but is generally performed to permit termination of pregnancy when a fetal abnormality is detected or to reassure parents when a fetus is unaffected. Pregnancies at risk of fetal abnormality may be identified in various ways. A pregnancy may be at increased risk because of advanced maternal age, because the couple already have an affected child, or because of a family history of a mendelian disorder or an inherited chromosomal rearrangement. Occasionally couples from certain ethnic groups whose pregnancies are at high risk of particular autosomal recessive disorders can be identified before the birth of an affected child by population screening programmes. In many mendelian disorders, particularly autosomal dominant disorders of late onset and X linked recessive disorders, family studies may be needed to assess the risk to the pregnancy and to determine the feasibility of prenatal diagnosis.

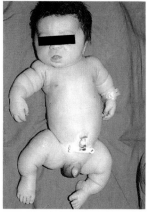 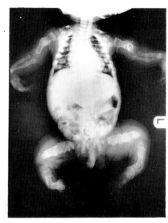

Osteogenesis imperfecta type II (perinatally lethal) can be detected by ultrasonography in second trimester.

Several important factors must be carefully considered before prenatal testing, one of which is the severity of the disorder. For many genetic diseases this is beyond doubt; some disorders lead inevitably to stillbirth or death in infancy or childhood. Perhaps more important, however, are conditions that result in children surviving with severe, multiple, and often progressive, physical and mental handicaps, such as Down's syndrome, neural tube defects, muscular dystrophy, and many of the multiple congenital malformation syndromes.

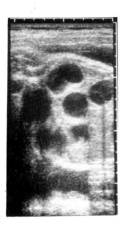

Prenatal detection of jejunal atresia indicating need for neonatal surgery.

The availability of treatment is also important to consider. When treatment is effective termination may not be appropriate and prenatal diagnosis is generally not indicated, unless early diagnosis permits more rapid institution of treatment, reducing illness, complications, and deaths. Phenylketonuria, for example, can be effectively treated after diagnosis in the neonatal period, and prenatal diagnosis, although possible for parents who already have an affected child, may be inappropriate. On the other hand, prenatal diagnosis of congenital malformations amenable to surgical correction is important as it allows the baby to be delivered in a unit with facilities for neonatal surgery and intensive care.

Applications of prenatal diagnosis

- Maternal serum
  screening — α fetoprotein estimation
- Ultrasonography — structural abnormalities
- Amniocentesis — α fetoprotein and
  acetylcholinesterase
  — chromosomal analysis
  — biochemical analysis
- Chorionic villus
  sampling — DNA analysis
  — chromosomal analysis
  — biochemical analysis
- Fetoscopy — direct examination
  — fetal sampling

A prenatal test must be sufficiently reliable to permit decisions about a pregnancy. Some conditions can be diagnosed with certainty, others cannot. For example, in mendelian disorders amenable to DNA analysis but for which specific gene probes are not available and the biochemical defect in the disorder is not known, the use of linked DNA markers allows a quantified risk to be given for a pregnancy.

As an abnormal result on prenatal testing may lead to termination this course of action must be acceptable to the couple. Careful assessment of their attitudes is important, and even those couples who clearly elect for termination need continued counselling and psychological support afterwards. Couples who do not contemplate termination may still request a prenatal diagnosis to help them to prepare for the outcome of the pregnancy, and these requests should not be dismissed.

Methods of prenatal diagnosis

Some causes of increased maternal serum α fetoprotein concentration

Underestimated gestational age

Threatened abortion

Multiple pregnancy

Fetal abnormality
  Anencephaly
  Open neural tube defect
  Anterior abdominal wall defect
  Turner's syndrome
  Bowel atresias
  Skin defects
Maternal hereditary persistence of α fetoprotein

Placental haemangioma

Screening of maternal serum

Testing of maternal serum has limited use for detecting genetic disease in the fetus but is valuable in screening for neural tube defects. About 80% of cases of open neural tube defects and over 90% of those of anencephaly can be detected by an increased maternal serum α fetoprotein concentration at 16-18 weeks' gestation. High concentrations indicate a need for further assessment. Screening of serum α fetoprotein alone is not sufficiently reliable in high risk cases in which a previous infant has been affected, and in these cases ultrasonography and amniocentesis should be offered.

A low serum α fetoprotein concentration indicates an increased risk of Down's syndrome. In future amniocentesis for chromosomal analysis may be offered on the basis of a composite risk estimated from the maternal age and the serum α fetoprotein, unconjugated oestriol, and human chorionic gonadotrophin concentrations. This would increase the detection rate of Down's syndrome without increasing the number of amnioceteses performed.

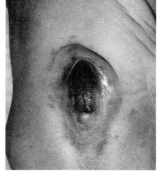

Lumbar meningomyelocele.

The possible identification of circulating trophoblast cells in maternal blood offers a potential method of detecting genetic disorders in the fetus. The application to prenatal diagnosis will, however, probably be limited as trophoblast cells are difficult to isolate and may represent cells arising from previous pregnancies.

Prenatal diagnosis

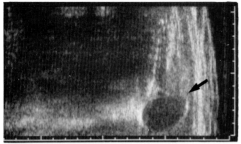

Large lumbosacral meningomyelocele.

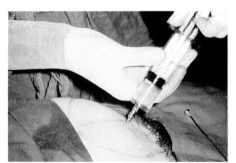

Shortened limb in Saldino-Noonan autosomal recessive bone dysplasia syndrome.

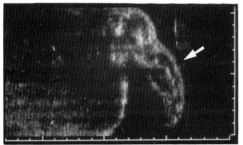

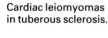
Cardiac leiomyomas in tuberous sclerosis.

Ultrasonography

Obstetric indications for ultrasonography are well established and include confirmation of viable pregnancy, assessment of gestational age, location of the placenta, and monitoring fetal growth. Ultrasonography is an integral part of amniocentesis, chorionic villus sampling, and fetoscopy and has an increasingly important role in prenatal diagnosis of structural abnormalities in the fetus as skill develops and scanners give higher resolution.

Disorders such as neural tube defects, severe skeletal dysplasias, and abnormalities of abdominal organs may all be detected by ultrasonography between 17 and 20 weeks' gestation, and hydrocephalus may be detected later in pregnancy. These abnormalities may be recognised during routine scanning of apparently normal pregnancies, and this allows the parents to be counselled about the abnormality and plans to be made for the neonatal management of disorders that are amenable to surgical correction. Centres specialising in high resolution ultrasonography can detect an increasing number of other abnormalities, such as structural abnormalities of the brain, various types of congenital heart disease, clefts of the lip and palate, and microphthalmia.

Most single congenital abnormalities follow multifactorial inheritance and carry a low risk of recurrence, but the safety of scanning provides an ideal method of screening subsequent pregnancies and usually gives reassurance about the normality of the fetus. Syndromes of multiple congenital abnormalities, however, may follow mendelian patterns of inheritance with high risks of recurrence; for many of these, ultrasonography is the only available method of prenatal diagnosis.

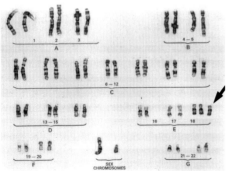

Amniocentesis procedure.

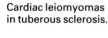

Trisomy 18 karyotype detected by analysis of cultured amniotic cells.

Amniocentesis

Amniocentesis—a well established and widely available method for prenatal diagnosis—is performed from 15 to 16 weeks' gestation. It is reliable and safe, causing an increased risk of miscarriage of around 0·5%. About 20 ml of amniotic fluid is aspirated directly, with or without local anaesthesia, after location of the placenta by ultrasonography. The fluid is normally clear and yellow and contains amniotic cells, which can be cultured. Contamination of the fluid with blood usually suggests puncture of the placenta and may hamper subsequent analysis. Discoloration of the fluid may suggest impending fetal death.

The main indications for amniocentesis are for estimating α fetoprotein concentration and acetylcholinesterase activity in amniotic fluid in pregnancies at increased risk of neural tube defects and for chromosomal analysis of cultured amniotic cells in those at increased risk of Down's syndrome associated with advanced maternal age. In specific cases biochemical analysis of amniotic fluid or cultured cells may be required for diagnosing inborn errors of metabolism. Tests on amniotic fluid usually yield results within 7-10 days whereas those requiring cultured cells may take around 3-4 weeks.

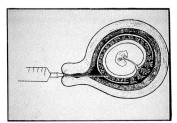

Procedure for transcervical chorionic villus sampling.

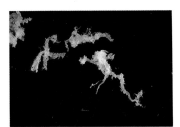

Chorionic villus material.

Chorionic villus sampling

Chorionic villus sampling is a recent technique in which fetally derived chorionic villus material is obtained transcervically with a flexible catheter between eight and 12 weeks' gestation or by transabdominal puncture and aspiration at any time up to term. Both methods are performed under ultrasonographic guidance, and fetal viability is checked before and after the procedure. The risk of miscarriage related to sampling in the first trimester in experienced hands is probably about 2% higher than the rate of spontaneous abortions at this time.

Dissection of fetal chorionic villus material from maternal decidua permits analysis of the fetal genotype. The main indications for chorionic villus sampling include the diagnosis of chromosomal disorders and an increasing number of inborn errors of metabolism and conditions amenable to DNA analysis. The advantage of this method of testing is the earlier timing of the procedure, which allows the result to be available by about 12 weeks' gestation, with earlier and easier termination of pregnancy, if required. These advantages are leading to an increased demand for the procedure in preference to amniocentesis, which has important consequences in planning services. If the availability of the procedure is limited, conditions that can be diagnosed only by this method must be given priority, together with high risk cases.

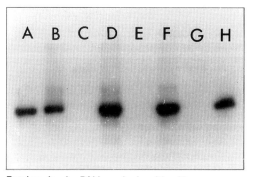

Fetal sexing by DNA analysis with a Y chromosome specific probe.
(Lanes A, B, H, control male; C, G, control female; E, mother; F, father; D, chorionic villus (male).)

To obtain a prenatal diagnosis in the first trimester it is important to identify high risk situations and counsel couples before pregnancy so that appropriate arrangements can be made and, when necessary, supplementary family studies organised.

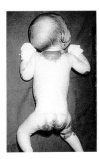

Lethal form of autosomal recessive epidermolysis bullosa can be diagnosed by fetal skin biopsy.

Fetoscopy

Fetoscopy is a highly specialised technique performed with a fibreoptic endoscope. The procedure is carried out in the second trimester in cases in which the fetus must be seen directly to identify dysmorphic features or to obtain fetal samples. It is possible to take fetal blood samples and skin biopsy specimens under direct ultrasonographic guidance without using an endoscope, and as the number of disorders amenable to DNA analysis increases and more tests can be performed on chorionic villus samples the indications for fetoscopy are decreasing.

Embryo biopsy

Preimplantation embryo biopsy is now technically feasible. In this method in vitro fertilisation and embryo culture would be followed by biopsy of one or two outer embryonal cells at the 8-16 cell stage of development. DNA analysis of a single cell and possibly chromosomal analysis of cultured cells could be performed so that only embryos free of a particular genetic defect would be reimplanted. This method may occasionally be more acceptable than other forms of prenatal diagnosis but the rate of successful pregnancies would be reduced.

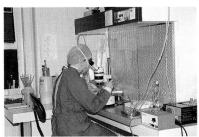

In vitro fertilisation laboratory.

Illustrations produced by kind permission were: the ultrasonographic scans of jejunal atresia, meningomyelocele, Saldino-Noonan syndrome, and cardiac leiomyomas, Dr Sylvia Rimmer; meningomyelocele, Dr Dian Donnai; the trisomy 18 karyotype, Dr Lorraine Gaunt; the chorionic villus maternal, Dr A Andrews; and the autoradiograph of fetal sexing, Mr R Mountford, St Mary's Hospital, Manchester.

TREATMENT OF GENETIC DISORDERS

Helen M Kingston

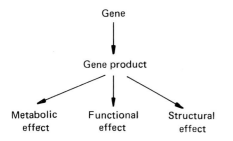

The prevention of inherited disease by means of genetic and reproductive counselling and prenatal diagnosis is often emphasised. Genetic disorders may, however, be amenable to treatment, either symptomatic or potentially curative. Treatment may range from conventional drug or dietary management and surgery to the future possibility of gene therapy. The level at which therapeutic intervention can be applied is influenced by the state of knowledge about the primary genetic defect, its effect, its interaction with environmental factors, and the way in which these may be modified.

Conventional treatment

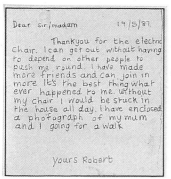

Letter written by boy aged 11 with Duchenne muscular dystrophy.

Increasing knowledge of the molecular and biochemical basis of genetic disorders leads to better prospects for therapeutic intervention and even the possibility of prenatal treatment in some disorders. The primary defect in many disorders, however, is not yet amenable to specific treatment. Conventional treatment aimed at relieving the symptoms and preventing complications remains important and may require a multidisciplinary approach. Management of Duchenne muscular dystrophy, for example, includes neurological and orthopaedic assessment and treatment, physiotherapy, treatment of chest infections and heart failure, mobility aids, home modifications, appropriate schooling, and support for the family, all of which aim at lessening the burden of the disorder. Lay organisations often provide additional support for the patients and their families; the Muscular Dystrophy Group, for example, employs family care officers, who work closely with families and the medical services.

Gene therapy

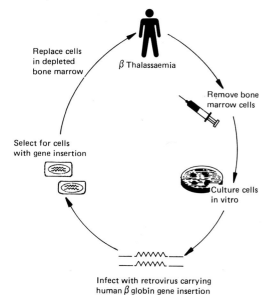

Potential strategy for gene therapy in β thalassaemia.

The prospect of curing genetic disorders with gene therapy is being investigated and has provoked much debate. In theory genetic disease could be cured by manipulating the genome directly to repair a genetic defect or by introducing a functioning donor gene into suitable recipient stem cells. Several experimental strategies have shown that gene transfer is possible. One method is to transfect host cells with retroviruses carrying donor DNA, but this is not yet a therapeutic option in human disease. To be successful the donor DNA needs to be stably incorporated into the host genome and expressed in a controlled manner at adequate levels in the correct cells. Dangers of insertional mutagenesis exist; an inserted donor gene might disrupt a host gene and replace one genetic disorder with another or increase the risk of neoplasia. There are ethical concerns about manipulating the human genome and especially about introducing foreign DNA into germline cells. If a genetic manipulation is not heritable, however, affected descendants will also require treatment.

Gene product replacement

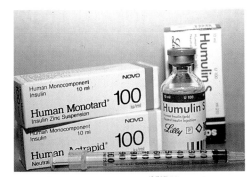
Insulins with human sequence prepared biosynthetically or by enzymatic modification of porcine material.

A simpler alternative to altering the genome is to replace a missing gene product. This strategy is effective when the gene product is a circulatory peptide or protein and is the standard treatment for haemophilia and growth hormone deficiency. The potential for direct replacement of missing intracellular enzymes is being determined experimentally. An alternative method of replacement is that of organ or cellular transplantation, which aims at providing a permanent functioning source of the missing gene product.

When the gene product is needed for metabolism within the central nervous system the blood-brain barrier presents an obstacle to systemic replacement treatment. Another potential problem is the initiation of an immunological reaction to the administered protein by the recipient. Successful production of human gene products, such as insulin and growth hormone, by recombinant DNA techniques may reduce this risk and will ensure adequate supplies for clinical use.

Metabolic manipulation

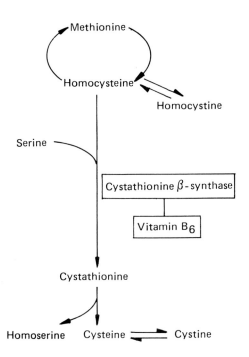
Pathway for homocysteine metabolism: most cases of homocystinuria are due to deficiency of cystathionine β-synthase, which requires vitamin B_6 cofactor.

Many inborn errors of metabolism due to enzyme deficiencies can be treated effectively. Although direct replacement of the missing enzyme is not generally possible, enzyme activity can be enhanced in some disorders. For example, phenobarbitone induces hepatic glucuronyl transferase activity and may lower circulating concentrations of unconjugated bilirubin in the Crigler-Najjar syndrome type 2. Vitamins act as cofactors in certain enzymatic reactions and can be effective if given in doses above the usual physiological requirements; homocystinuria may respond to treatment with vitamin B_6, certain types of methylmalonic aciduria to vitamin B_{12}, and multiple carboxylase deficiency to biotin. It may also be possible to stimulate alternate metabolic pathways; thiamine may permit a switch to pyruvate metabolism by means of pyruvate dehydrogenase in pyruvate carboxylase deficiency.

The clinical features of an inborn error of metabolism may be due to accumulation of a substrate that cannot be metabolised. The classical example is phenylketonuria, in which the absence of phenylalanine hydroxylase results in high concentrations of phenylalanine, causing mental retardation, seizures, and eczema. The treatment consists of limiting dietary intake of phenylalanine to that essential for normal growth. Galactosaemia is similarly treated by a galactose free diet. In other disorders the harmful substrate may have to be removed by alternative means, such as the chelation of copper with penicillamine in Wilson's disease and peritoneal dialysis or haemodialysis in certain disorders of organic acid metabolism. In hyperuricaemia urate excretion may be enhanced by probenecid or its production inhibited by allopurinol, an inhibitor of xanthine oxidase.

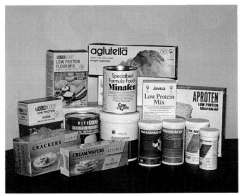
Products low in phenylalanine used in dietary management of phenylketonuria.

In another group of inborn errors of metabolism the signs and symptoms are due to deficiency of an end product of a metabolic reaction, and treatment depends on replacing this end product. Defects occurring at different stages in biosynthesis of adrenocortical steroids in the various forms of congenital adrenal hyperplasia are treated by replacing cortisol, alone or together with aldosterone in the salt losing form. Congenital hypothyroidism can similarly be treated with thyroxine replacement. In some disorders, such as oculocutaneous albinism in which a deficiency in melanin production occurs, replacing the end product of the metabolic pathway is, however, not possible.

Environmental modification

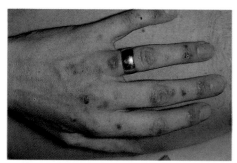

Porphyria cutanea tarda.

The effects of some genetic disorders may be minimised by avoiding known environmental triggers. Certain drugs will precipitate attacks in porphyria, including anticonvulsants, oestrogens, barbiturates, and sulphonamides in acute intermittent porphyria and oestrogens and alcohol in porphyria cutanea tarda. Other drugs, such as primaquine and dapsone, as well as ingesting fava beans cause haemolysis in glucose-6-phosphate dehydrogenase deficiency. Suxamethonium must not be given to people with pseudocholinesterase deficiency, and risks are associated with anaesthesia in myotonic dystrophy.

Exposure to sunlight precipitates skin fragility and blistering in all the porphyrias except the acute intermittent form. Sunlight should also be avoided in xeroderma pigmentosum (a rare defect of DNA repair) and in oculocutaneous albinism because of the increased risk of skin cancer.

Surgical management

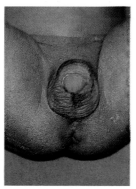

Virilisation of female genitalia in congenital adrenal hyperplasia (21-hydroxylase deficiency).

Surgery plays an important part in various genetic disorders, not only those concerning primary congenital malformations. Virilisation of the external genitalia in girls with congenital adrenal hyperplasia is secondary to excess production of androgenic steroids in utero and requires reconstructive surgery. In some disorders structural complications may occur later, such as the aortic dilatation that may develop in Marfan's syndrome. Surgery may also be needed in genetic disorders that predispose to neoplasia, such as the multiple endocrine neoplasia syndromes, and screening family members at risk permits early intervention and improves prognosis. Occasionally malformations detected during pregnancy, such as posterior urethral valves, may be amenable to prenatal surgical intervention.

The letter was reproduced by kind permission of Robert Little; the illustration of porphyria cutanea tarda by kind permission of Dr T Kingston, Skin Hospital, Salford; and that of congenital adrenal hyperplasia by kind permission of Dr Dian Donnai, St Mary's Hospital, Manchester.

GENE STRUCTURE AND FUNCTION

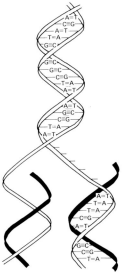

The DNA molecule is fundamental to cell metabolism and cell division as well as providing the basis for inherited characteristics. Nucleic acid, initially called nuclein, was discovered by Friedrich Miescher in 1869, but it was not until 1953 that Watson and Crick produced their model for the double helical structure of DNA and proposed the mechanism for DNA replication. During the 1960s the genetic code was found to reside in the sequence of nucleotides comprising the DNA molecule, a group of three nucleotides coding for an amino acid. The rapid expansion of molecular techniques in the past decade has led to a better understanding of human genetic disease. The structure and function of many genes has been elucidated, and determining the nucleotide sequence of an entire gene is possible. The molecular pathology underlying various disorders is now defined, and DNA analysis can be used for investigating affected families.

DNA structure

Genetic code (RNA)*

First base (5′ end)	Second base				Third base (3′ end)
	U	C	A	G	
U	Phe	Ser	Tyr	Cys	U
	Phe	Ser	Tyr	Cys	C
	Leu	Ser	Stop	Stop	A
	Leu	Ser	Stop	Trp	G
C	Leu	Pro	His	Arg	U
	Leu	Pro	His	Arg	C
	Leu	Pro	Gln	Arg	A
	Leu	Pro	Gln	Arg	G
A	Ile	Thr	Asn	Ser	U
	Ile	Thr	Asn	Ser	C
	Ile	Thr	Lys	Arg	A
	Met	Thr	Lys	Arg	G
G	Val	Ala	Asp	Gly	U
	Val	Ala	Asp	Gly	C
	Val	Ala	Glu	Gly	A
	Val	Ala	Glu	Gly	G

*Uracil (U) replaces thymine (T) in RNA.

A single strand of DNA consists of a backbone of deoxyribose sugar units linked by phosphate groups. The orientation of the phosphate groups defines the 5′ and 3′ ends of the molecule. The purine bases adenine (A) and guanine (G) and the pyrimidine bases cytosine (C) and thymine (T) are attached to the deoxyribose units, and their sequence along the molecule constitutes the genetic code. The coding unit, or codon, consists of three nucleotide bases; for example, on the DNA sense strand the codon TTC codes for phenylalanine and AGA for arginine; the triplet ATG codes for methionine and also acts as a signal to start protein synthesis on messenger RNA (mRNA); in addition, three triplets (TAA, TAG, and TGA) act as termination signals. As the four bases give 64 possible codon combinations and there are only 20 amino acids most amino acids are specified by at least two codons and the code is said to be degenerate. The DNA code is universal to all organisms with the exception of mitochondrial DNA, which has slightly different codons.

In the nucleus DNA exists as a double stranded helix in which the order of the bases on one strand is complementary to that on the other. The bases are held together by hydrogen bonds, which allow the strands to separate and rejoin. Adenine is always paired with thymine and cytosine with guanine. This specific pairing is fundamental to DNA replication, during which the two DNA strands separate and each acts as a template for the synthesis of a new strand. The genetic code is therefore maintained during cell division, and as each cell contains an existing and a newly synthesised strand of DNA the process is called semiconservative replication. A damaged DNA strand may be repaired and reconstituted in a similar way.

DNA molecule comprising sugar and phosphate backbone and paired nucleotides joined by hydrogen bonds.

Gene structure and function

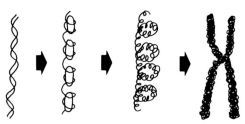

Diagrammatic representation of packaging of DNA into chromosome structure.

Each human somatic cell contains 6×10^9 base pairs of DNA, which is equivalent to about 2m of linear DNA. Packaging of the DNA is achieved by the double helix being coiled around histone proteins to form nucleosomes and then condensed by further coiling into the chromosome structure seen at metaphase. A single cell does not express all of its genes, and active genes are packaged into a more accessible chromatin configuration, which allows them to be transcribed. Some genes are expressed at low levels in all cells and are called housekeeping genes, others are tissue specific and expressed only in certain tissues or cell types.

An estimated 50 000-100 000 pairs of functional genes exist in humans, yet these constitute only a small proportion of total genomic DNA. More than 90% of the genome consists of non-coding DNA, whose function is not clearly defined. Much of this DNA has a unique sequence, but between 30% and 40% consists of repetitive sequences that may be dispersed throughout the genome or arranged as regions of tandem repeats, known as satellite DNA. In tandem repeats the number of times that the core sequence is repeated varies among different people, and this gives rise to hypervariable regions.

The enormous variation occurring in non-coding DNA among different subjects is illustrated particularly well in certain hypervariable minisatellite regions throughout the genome that share a short common core sequence in their variable number of tandem repeats (VNTRs). These hypervariable minisatellite regions are stably inherited and give a pattern of DNA fragments of various sizes on analysis that is unique to each person, forming the basis of the DNA fingerprinting test.

Other DNA variations due to differences in nucleotide sequence that occur close to genes of interest can be used to track genes through families using DNA probes; this approach has revolutionised the predictive tests available for mendelian disorders such as Duchenne muscular dystrophy and cystic fibrosis.

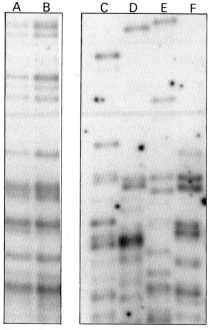

Part of fingerprinting autoradiograph showing bands detected by minisatellite DNA probe in blood samples from monozygous twins (A and B) who have identical bands and four unrelated subjects (C-F) who have different bands.

Transcription and translation

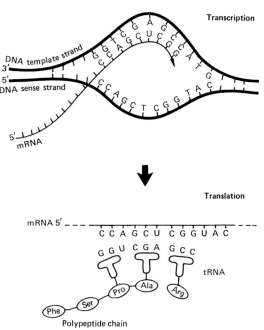

Process of transcription and translation.

The genetic code carried by DNA is translated into a protein product by means of RNA molecules. The structure of mRNA is similar to that of DNA, except that the sugar backbone is composed of ribose and uracil (U) replaces thymine (T) as one of the bases. One strand of the DNA acts as a template for mRNA synthesis, a process that occurs by pairing of specific bases as it does in DNA synthesis. In experimental systems the reverse of this reaction—the synthesis of complementary DNA (cDNA) using mRNA as a template—is possible with the enzyme reverse transcriptase. This has proved to be an immensely valuable procedure for investigating human genetic disorders as it allows cDNA probes to be produced that correspond exactly to the coding sequence of a human gene.

Messenger RNA is translated into protein in the cytoplasm in association with ribosomes and transfer RNAs (tRNAs). Each tRNA molecule binds a specific amino acid and has three bases forming an anticodon triplet that allows it to bind to a complementary mRNA codon, starting with the initiation signal AUG. Peptide bonds form between the amino acids as the tRNAs are aligned on the ribosome until a stop codon on the mRNA is reached. Several ribosomes associate with each mRNA strand, forming polysomes, thus permitting simultaneous production of several polypeptide chains from one mRNA molecule. The active three dimensional configuration of proteins such as insulin and the collagens is achieved by post-translational modification. Alternative methods of processing and splicing mRNA in certain circumstances permits the production of different protein products from some genes. Gene rearrangement may also occur; rearrangement of the immunoglobulin genes in lymphocytes, for example, is responsible for the enormous structural diversity of antibodies.

Gene structure and function

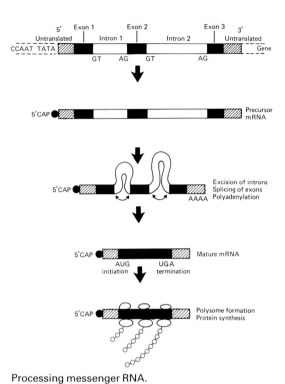

Processing messenger RNA.

The fingerprinting autoradiograph was reproduced by kind permission of Dr A Read, St Mary's Hospital, Manchester.

The coding sequence of a gene is not continuous but is interrupted by varying numbers and lengths of intervening non-coding sequences whose function, if any, is not known. The coding sequences are called exons and the intervening sequences introns. The size and complexity of human genes varies, the largest so far identified is the dystrophin gene, which causes Duchenne muscular dystrophy when it is defective and spans two million base pairs with 14 000 bases of coding sequence distributed among at least 60 exons.

In addition to the introns, there are non-coding regions of DNA at both 5′ and 3′ ends of genes. There are also regulatory sequences that occur in and around the gene that control its function. In the 5′ flanking region two conserved, or consensus, sequences known as the TATA box and the CAT box, are concerned with controlling mRNA transcription. Methylation of cytosine nucleotides plays a part in regulating gene activity, and enhancer sequences may also be involved, as well as more distant regulatory elements.

Both coding and non-coding DNA sequences in a gene are initially transcribed into mRNA. The sequences corresponding to the introns are then cut out and the exons spliced together to produce mature mRNA. Conserved sequences at the splicing sites enables their recognition in this complex process. Other modifications include the addition of a cap structure at the 5′ end of the mRNA molecule and polyadenylation at the 3′ end.

A genetic mutation may have its effect at any stage in the process of transcription or translation, producing mRNA that is unstable or that cannot be translated into a functional polypeptide. Many different types of mutation are recognised in human genetic disorders, including point mutations, deletions, insertions, rearrangements, and duplications. In different families with the same genetic condition the mutation causing the disorder is not always the same; β thalassaemia, for example, may be due to any of these mutations.

Mutations have a wide range of effects. Point mutations, for example, may cause amino acid substitution; disrupt a promotor sequence; alter an initiator codon; generate a terminator codon; or change the codon at a splicing site. Deletions may remove a substantial part of the gene or may alter the reading frame if the number of bases deleted is not a multiple of three, and this has a catastrophic effect on protein synthesis. For example, a deletion in the dystrophin gene that causes a frame shift results in Duchenne muscular dystrophy, whereas one that does not change the reading frame results in the milder Becker's muscular dystrophy.

TECHNIQUES OF DNA ANALYSIS

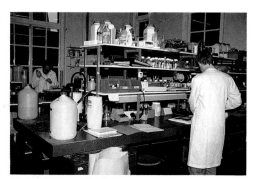

Molecular genetics laboratory.

DNA analysis is becoming a standard investigation in an increasing number of mendelian disorders. The genetic state of family members and pregnancies at risk can be determined in many conditions, including the haemoglobinopathies, Duchenne muscular dystrophy, cystic fibrosis, and Huntington's chorea. The index case is generally diagnosed by means of conventional investigations, such as electrophoresis of haemoglobin in thalassaemia and muscle biopsy in Duchenne muscular dystrophy. DNA studies may clarify the diagnosis in disorders that are associated with specific mutations or gene deletions. The main impact of DNA analysis in clinical practice has been in detecting carriers of X linked recessive disorders, in presymptomatic diagnosis of autosomal dominant disorders, and in prenatal diagnosis of all categories of mendelian disorders. This chapter summarises the standard techniques of DNA analysis that are used in the clinical investigation of affected families. In several health authority regions and health boards throughout the United Kingdom molecular genetics laboratories are associated with departments of clinical genetics and provide DNA analysis as a service to families with particular genetic disorders.

DNA extraction

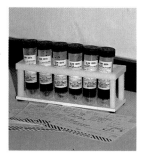

DNA can be extracted from 10-20 ml whole blood.

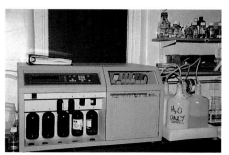

Automated DNA extraction.

DNA can be extracted by using standard techniques from any tissue containing nucleated cells, including blood and chorionic villus material. Once extracted, the DNA is stable and can be stored indefinitely so that samples from people with genetic disorders can be collected and saved for the future investigation of other family members. Storing samples has already benefited many families whose elderly or affected relatives were no longer living when DNA testing became possible, yet from whom samples were needed to interpret predictive tests.

Restriction enzymes

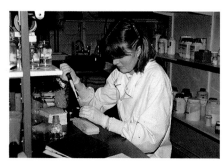

Preparing restriction enzyme digest reaction.

```
C C C G G G

G G G C C C

       Sma I

C T G C A G

G A C G T C

  Pst I
```

Recognition sequences of two restriction enzymes.

The discovery of bacterial restriction enzymes in 1969 has been important in developing techniques to analyse human DNA. Restriction enzymes recognise specific DNA sequences and cleave double stranded DNA at these sites. Each enzyme has its own recognition sequence and will cut genomic DNA into a series of fragments that can then be analysed. The size of the fragments produced is constant in an individual subject but commonly varies among subjects because of differences in non-coding DNA sequences. This variation forms the basis of some predictive tests, which are discussed later.

Electrophoresis

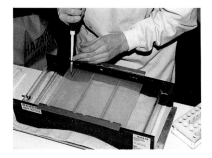

Loading digested DNA samples on to agarose gel.

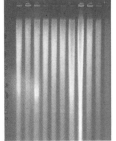

DNA fragments in gel after electrophoresis stained with ethidium bromide and viewed under ultraviolet light.

The DNA fragments produced by cutting genomic DNA with restriction enzymes can be ordered according to their size by electrophoresis in an agarose gel. The small fragments migrate faster down the gel than the larger ones, giving a track of DNA fragments of progressively diminishing size. The length of a particular fragment can be determined from the distance of its migration in the gel with reference to marker fragments of known size.

Southern blotting

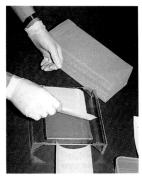

Setting up Southern blot: placing filter on to agarose gel.

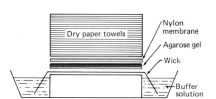

The DNA fragments in a gel are denatured into single strands and transferred by the technique of Southern blotting on to a nitrocellulose filter or nylon membrane. Fluid rising through the gel transfers the DNA on to the membrane, retaining the alignment of the fragments. Although conventionally performed with a reservoir of buffer solution, the procedure may also be performed without buffer as fluid absorbed directly from the gel by the paper towels is sufficient to permit transfer of the DNA. The DNA binds to the membrane, providing a stable array of DNA fragments that can be analysed by mixing with a DNA probe in a hybridisation reaction. The basis of this reaction is the ability of complementary DNA strands to bind together.

DNA probe hybridisation

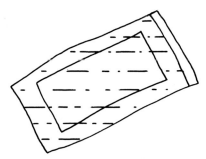

Radiolabelling DNA probe with phosphorus-32.

A probe is a piece of single stranded DNA, radiolabelled with phosphorus-32, which is used to detect homologous sequences in a sample of genomic DNA. Probes used to study mendelian disorders represent unique sequences that occur only once in the genome and may correspond to the gene of interest, to flanking DNA, or to more distant DNA sequences. Gene specific probes derived from genomic DNA contain both coding and non-coding sequences. Complementary DNA (cDNA) probes are synthesised from the messenger RNA of the gene under study with reverse transcriptase and contain only coding sequences. Oligonucleotide probes, containing around 19 nucleotides, can be synthesised for a specific region of a gene whose sequence is known. Randomly generated probes do not correspond to specific genes but can be used to study families if they are shown to be located close to a gene of interest.

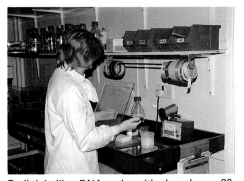

Membrane washed in solution containing radioactive DNA probe during hybridisation reaction.

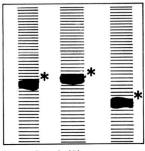

Dense bands (*) on autoradiography indicating hybridisation of probe DNA to homologous sequence in sample DNA.

Probes are prepared by cloning the sequence of interest with recombinant DNA techniques. The DNA fragment to be used as a probe is incorporated into vector DNA, usually a bacterial plasmid. The recombinant vector plasmid is then amplified in *Escherichia coli*, allowing large quantities of the probe DNA to be retrieved. The probe is radiolabelled and added to a solution for hybridisation with a membrane blotted with the patient's DNA. The single stranded DNA probe will bind to any DNA fragment on the membrane that has a matching DNA sequence. These fragments can be identified as visible bands in an *x* ray film placed in contact with the membrane (autoradiography).

Application to genetic disorders

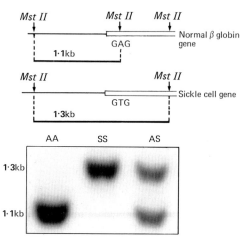

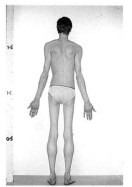

Autoradiograph showing detection of sickle cell mutation by altered size of DNA fragments produced by cleavage with *Mst II* restriction enzyme.

Becker's muscular dystrophy: proximal muscle wasting, winging of scapulae, and pseudohypertrophy of calf and deltoid muscles.

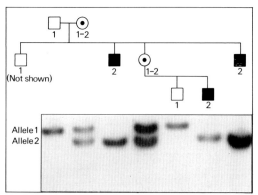

Autoradiograph showing restriction fragment length polymorphism (alleles 1 and 2) detected by X chromosomal DNA probe linked to gene for Becker's muscular dystrophy: disease gene segregates with maternal allele 2, providing a marker for the disorder, subject to recombination.

Deletions

Disorders due to gene deletions can be detected directly by the absence of specific DNA bands on an autoradiograph if gene specific probes are available. α Thalassaemia and some cases of β thalassaemia, haemophilia A, and Duchenne muscular dystrophy, for example, can be identified in this way.

Point mutations

Genetic disorders due to point mutations are amenable to direct detection if the mutation affects a recognition site for a restriction enzyme or if specific oligonucleotide probes are available. In sickle cell disease a point mutation changes the codon GAG to GTG in the β globin gene and results in the substitution of valine for glutamic acid in haemoglobin. The mutation alters the recognition site of the restriction enzyme *Mst II*, changing the size of the DNA fragment detected by the β globin gene probe on autoradiography. An alternative method of testing for sickle cell disease or its carrier state is to use oligonucleotide probes corresponding to the normal and mutant β globin gene sequences. Each oligonucleotide probe will bind only to its specific genomic counterpart, so that the HbA probe gives an autoradiographic band only with the normal β globin gene, and the HbS probe gives a band only with the mutant β globin gene. Both probes will hybridise with the DNA from heterozygous subjects.

Restriction fragment length polymorphisms (RFLPs)

When a mutation causing a genetic disorder cannot be detected directly prediction of genetic state in a person may still be possible by identifying other genetic variations (polymorphisms) that can be tracked through the family. Variations in non-coding DNA sequences are extremely frequent throughout the genome, and when they affect restriction enzyme cleavage sites DNA fragments of different sizes will result from restriction endonuclease digestion of the DNA. These variations are called restriction fragment length polymorphisms (RFLPs) and can be used as markers for genetic disorders if they occur in or near a gene of interest. Before prediction is possible a family must have DNA analysis performed to see if there is a variation in the size of fragments detected by an appropriate probe that gives an informative pattern in the family. The particular fragment associated with the disease gene must then be identified so that it can be looked for in the relative or pregnancy being tested.

When a DNA variation occurring within or very close to a gene is detected by a gene specific probe, prediction by analysis of RFLPs will usually determine the genetic state with near certainty, as in haemophilia A. Occasionally a gene is so large (as in Duchenne muscular dystrophy) that the disease mutation and a marker variation within the gene may be sufficiently far apart for recombination to occur between the two sites at meiosis, and there will be a small error in predicting genetic state from RFLP analysis. In disorders such as Huntington's chorea and cystic fibrosis, in which the genes responsible have not yet been cloned, RFLP analysis makes use of DNA polymorphisms shown to be in close proximity to the disease gene by family studies. These markers are said to be linked to the disease gene if they cosegregate in affected families. The closer the DNA marker sequence is to the disease gene the less likely it is to segregate independently because of recombination and the greater the accuracy of predicting genetic state from the marker pattern. In practice markers which show less than 5% recombination with a disease gene are useful in detecting carriers and in prenatal diagnosis. As 1% recombination occurs between loci that are separated by around one million base pairs these markers may be up to five million bases away from the gene being studied.

New techniques

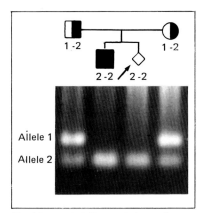

Allele 1
Allele 2

Rapid prenatal diagnosis in cystic fibrosis using polymerase chain reaction: fetus (↗) has inherited same parental alleles as affected sibling, indicating that it is also affected.

New techniques of DNA analysis are continually being developed which have an appreciable impact on the clinical investigation of genetic disease. The polymerase chain reaction and pulsed field gel electrophoresis are two such examples.

In the polymerase chain reaction oligonucleotide primers corresponding to sequences at each end of a DNA region of interest are synthesised. With the primers this region can be amplified in a sample of genomic DNA—for example, chorionic villus DNA—by successive rounds of replication with DNA polymerase. The amplified segment produced by the polymerase chain reaction is then cut with the appropriate restriction enzyme, run in an agarose gel, and detected directly under ultraviolet light after staining with ethidium bromide. The technique permits rapid analysis of DNA, giving results within one to two days after sampling, compared with seven to 10 days by conventional analysis. This is particularly helpful when performing prenatal diagnosis.

Pulsed field gel electrophoresis permits the separation of large fragments of DNA. The technique is being used for long range mapping of the genome and facilitates identification of gene deletions causing genetic disorders.

The illustration of the polymerase chain reaction in prenatal diagnosis of cystic fibrosis was reproduced by kind permission of Mr A Ivinson, regional molecular genetics laboratory, St Mary's Hospital, Manchester, and that of Becker's muscular dystrophy by kind permission of Dr K Cumming, Withington Hospital, Manchester.

DNA ANALYSIS IN GENETIC DISORDERS

Examples of mapped autosomal genes

Disorder	Chromosome No
Porphyria cutanea tarda	1
Gaucher's disease	1
von Hippel-Lindau disease	3
Huntington's chorea	4
Polyposis coli	5
Haemochromatosis	6
21-Hydroxylase deficiency	6
Osteogenesis imperfecta (some forms)	7
Cystic fibrosis	7
Galactosaemia	9
Multiple endocrine neoplasia IIa	10
Sickle cell anaemia and β thalassaemia	11
Acute intermittent porphyria	11
Phenylketonuria (classic)	12
Wilson's disease	13
Retinoblastoma	13
α₁-Antitrypsin deficiency	14
Tay-Sachs disease	15
α Thalassaemia	16
Adult polycystic kidney disease	16
Neurofibromatosis (peripheral)	17
Osteogenesis imperfecta (some forms)	17
Familial hypercholesterolaemia	19
Myotonic dystrophy	19
Alzheimer's disease (familial)	21
Homocystinuria	21
Hurler's syndrome (mucopolysaccharidosis I)	22
Neurofibromatosis (central)	22

The ability to analyse DNA has had an important impact on our understanding of genetic disorders. Many genes have now been cloned and sequenced and the mutations that cause disease identified. Many other genetic disorders, for which the genes are not yet isolated, have been mapped to particular chromosomal locations, and this permits predictive testing with linked DNA markers. It has been estimated that the entire human genome will be mapped and all the important genes sequenced by the end of the century. This is not unrealistic and promises to be of enormous benefit to families with genetic disorders and to potential gene carriers.

International meetings on human gene mapping, inaugurated in 1973, are held every two years and mark current progress. At the first meeting the total number of autosomal genes whose chromosomal location had been identified was 64. The corresponding number of mapped genes had risen to 928 by the ninth meeting in 1987. This tremendous increase reflects the addition of various molecular biological approaches to those of more traditional somatic cell genetics. The total number of mapped X linked loci has also risen, from 155 in 1973 to 308 in 1987. Single copy anonymous DNA segments, which may be used as DNA markers for genetic disorders, number more than 1500 for autosomes and over 300 for the X chromosome. Many of these are clinically useful probes that can be applied both to detecting carriers and to prenatal diagnosis.

In this concluding article some of the ways in which molecular techniques can be applied clinically are illustrated with selected genetic disorders as examples. In most genetic conditions amenable to prenatal diagnosis by DNA analysis studies must be performed on the family first to determine whether there is a DNA variation that gives an informative pattern, and certain key relatives must be available for testing to make prediction possible. Because chorionic villus sampling is performed at eight to nine weeks of gestation counselling and investigating a family before pregnancy is important to ensure that a couple have time to make fully informed decisions.

Haemoglobinopathies

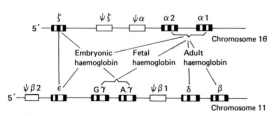

Globin gene clusters on chromosomes 11 and 16. (ψ denotes pseudogenes.)

The haemoglobinopathies constitute the most common autosomal disorders world wide and have profound effects on the provision of health care in some developing countries. They were among the first disorders to be analysed at a molecular DNA level, partly because the structure of haemoglobin was already well defined and also because fairly pure messenger RNA could be extracted from reticulocytes and used to produce complementary DNA probes. The globin gene clusters on chromosome 16 include two α globin genes and on chromosome 11 a β globin gene.

Various mutations in the β globin gene cause structural alterations in haemoglobin, the most important being the point mutation that produces haemoglobin S and causes sickle cell anaemia. Direct detection of the point mutation (described in the previous chapter) permits early prenatal diagnosis by analysis of DNA extracted from chorionic villus material.

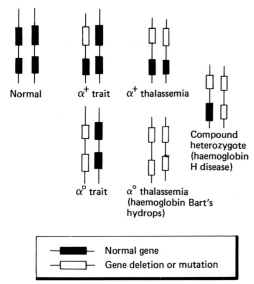

Representation of globin genes in various forms of α thalassaemia.

Normal
α⁺ trait
α⁺ thalassemia
α° trait
α° thalassaemia (haemoglobin Bart's hydrops)
Compound heterozygote (haemoglobin H disease)

━■━ Normal gene
━□━ Gene deletion or mutation

The thalassaemias are due to a reduced rate of production of one or more globin chains, leading to an imbalance in their production. In α thalassaemia production of α globin chains may be absent (α^0) or reduced (α^+). In the α^0 thalassaemia trait both α globin genes are deleted from one chromosome and in the homozygous state all four genes are deleted. In the α^+ thalassaemia trait only one α globin gene is inactivated, either by deletion or mutation, and the other is intact. Deleted genes can be detected directly in the homozygous state by failure of hybridisation with α globin gene probes.

In β thalassaemia over 30 different mutations causing the disorder have been identified, which result in β^0 and β^+ types depending on whether the production of β globin chains is absent or reduced. Major gene deletions are unusual in β thalassaemia, and most mutations entail point mutations or small deletions or insertions. To offer prenatal diagnosis by DNA analysis each individual family must be studied to determine the nature of the mutation. Particular mutations are common in certain populations, and specific oligonucleotide probes are available for prenatal diagnosis in many cases.

Cystic fibrosis

Cystic fibrosis is the commonest autosomal recessive disorder in northern Europeans and remains incurable, although survival is improved with supportive treatment. Detection of carriers in the population may soon be possible, but at present prevention depends largely on prenatal diagnosis being offered to couples who already have an affected child. The Brock test has been available for several years and predicts the likelihood of cystic fibrosis in a fetus at high risk by measuring enzyme activities of the microvilli in amniotic fluid. Early prenatal diagnosis is now possible by DNA analysis of chorionic villus material.

The cystic fibrosis gene has not yet been isolated, but family studies localised it to chromosome 7 in 1985. Several identified DNA probes that are closely linked to the cystic fibrosis locus on either side of the gene can be used clinically. An informative DNA pattern in a family is one in which the parental chromosomes carrying the cystic fibrosis gene can be identified from the DNA pattern in the affected child. The genetic state of a fetus depends on whether it shares one, two, or no haplotypes with the affected sibling. With currently available probes most families are informative for this type of prenatal diagnosis with a high degree of accuracy (99%). DNA analysis can similarly be used in families with cystic fibrosis to assess carrier state in healthy siblings. The likelihood of an unrelated spouse being a carrier can also be calculated because most chromosomes carrying the cystic fibrosis gene in northern Europeans carry a particular set of marker types that are uncommon in normal chromosomes. This linkage disequilibrium between the marker haplotype and the cystic fibrosis gene has no direct connection with the cystic fibrosis mutation but probably reflects the fact that most chromosomes carrying the gene are descended from a single ancestral mutant.

A healthy sibling of a patient with cystic fibrosis with an unrelated spouse has a fairly low risk of cystic fibrosis occurring in his or her children ($\frac{2}{3} \times \frac{1}{20} \times \frac{1}{4} = \frac{1}{120}$) and may find this reassuring. Analysis of DNA haplotypes might change the risk such that it becomes particularly high or particularly low, and this might influence decisions about reproduction and prenatal diagnosis. If the risk increases, however, but not to a level at which prenatal diagnosis becomes sufficiently reliable, parental anxiety will only be heightened. More certain detection of gene carriers in the general population will probably become feasible once the gene for cystic fibrosis has been isolated, and such couples may choose to defer tests until this is possible.

A   B   C   D

Allele 1

Allele 2

Autoradiographic bands detected by probe pJ311 in DNA digested with *Msp I* restriction endonuclease in family with cystic fibrosis. Affected child (lane B) is homozygous for allele 1, identifying the parental chromosomes that carry the cystic fibrosis gene. The fetus (lane C) has inherited one normal chromosome and one carrying the cystic fibrosis gene and is predicted to be a healthy carrier.

DNA analysis in genetic disorders

Huntington's chorea

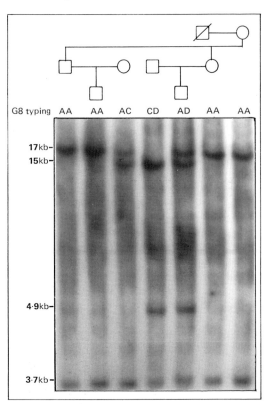

Inheritance of G8 haplotypes in DNA digested with *Hind III* restriction endonuclease (A=17, 3·7 kilobases (kb); B=17, 4·9 kb (not shown); C=15, 3·7 kb; and D=15, 4·9 kb).

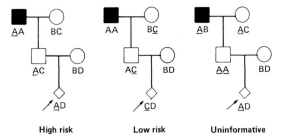

High risk   Low risk   Uninformative

Examples of fetal exclusion test results in Huntington's chorea.

Huntington's chorea is an autosomal dominant condition and is one of the most devastating genetic disorders, with the onset of involuntary movements and dementia being variable but commonly occurring between the ages of 35 and 55. The gene has not yet been cloned but was found to be linked to a probe called G8 in family studies in 1983, which localised the gene to the short arm of chromosome 4. The G8 probe detects polymorphisms with the restriction enzyme *Hind III*, and the four haplotypes, designated A, B, C, and D, can be tracked through affected families. Other linked probes are also now available and predictive testing for a person at risk is possible if the family structure is suitable and the marker pattern in the family is informative. People at risk, however, may not want predictive testing in the absence of any effective treatment. The potential for predictive testing raises many important ethical issues. Careful counselling before and after such tests is essential to ensure that the patient can cope with possible bad news from a test.

A major concern of many people at risk of developing the disease is that they may transmit the disorder to their children. A prenatal test can be performed that indicates the risk to a fetus without predicting the genetic state of the parent. The principle of the test is that it determines whether the fetus has inherited a chromosome from the affected or unaffected grandparent through the parent at risk. A chromosome from the affected grandparent confers a 50% risk (the same as the risk to the parent). A chromosome inherited from the unaffected grandparent reduces the risk to that associated with the chance of recombination having occurred between the gene for the disease and the probe being used. One potential problem with this type of test is that if a pregnancy identified as being at 50% risk continues to term and the parent subsequently develops Huntington's chorea this indicates that the child has probably also inherited the gene and will develop the disorder.

Duchenne muscular dystrophy

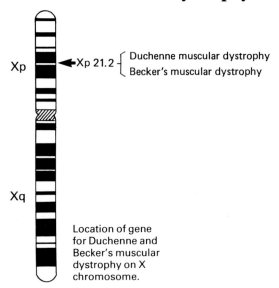

Location of gene for Duchenne and Becker's muscular dystrophy on X chromosome.

Duchenne muscular dystrophy was first described in 1861 and the X linked pattern of inheritance reported in 1943. A milder form of X linked muscular dystrophy identified by Becker in 1955 is now known to be due to a defect in the same gene. Duchenne muscular dystrophy has been reported in girls who have one X chromosome disrupted by a translocation between it and an autosome, with the normal X chromosome being preferentially inactivated. The site of the breakpoint in the cases of the chromosomal translocation is always located in the Xp21 band, which suggested that this was the location of the Duchenne gene. DNA probes identified from this region were shown to be linked to Duchenne muscular dystrophy in family studies in 1983, confirming this localisation. Other probes showing closer linkage have subsequently been identified and used in detecting carriers. Strategies were then devised to obtain DNA probes from within the gene by using DNA from a patient with a chromosomal deletion and from another with a chromosomal translocation. The gene that causes Duchenne and Becker's muscular dystrophy when it is defective has since been cloned and the gene product, dystrophin, identified. Several genomic and complementary DNA probes are now available for use in carrier detection and prenatal diagnosis.

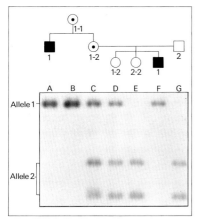

Restriction fragment length polymorphism (alleles 1 and 2) on X chromosome detected by probe pERT 87-15 in DNA digested with *Xmn* I restriction endonuclease. Dystrophy gene segregates with maternal allele 1, indicating that one daughter (lane D) is at high risk of being a carrier and the other (lane E) is at low risk.

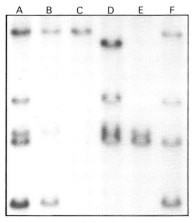

Autoradiographic bands corresponding to exons of dystrophin gene detected by probe Cf56 in DNA digested with *Pst* I restriction endonuclease from boys with Duchenne muscular dystrophy. Lane A: five exons with no deletion; lanes B-F: various exons deleted; lane D: also shows alteration in size of largest exon.

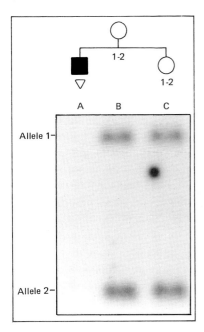

Restriction fragment length polymorphism and deletion detected with probe p20 in DNA digested with *Msp* I restriction endonuclease. (See text for interpretation.)
▽ = Deletion.

Several probes detect restriction fragment length polymorphisms (RFLPs) within the dystrophin gene. The variant bands identified on autoradiography can be used to track the disease gene through a family and make predictions about genetic state in female relatives and male fetuses at risk. As the dystrophin gene is so large (consisting of two million base pairs) and mutations causing muscular dystrophy may occur throughout the gene the gene mutation in a particular family may be a considerable distance from the RFLP site detected by the probe. Recombination between the two sites during gametogenesis may separate the loci so that absolute prediction about transmission of the mutation from parent to child cannot be made from RFLP studies. In family studies 5% recombination is observed and the prediction of genetic state can therefore be made with 95% accuracy.

About 60-70% of males with Duchenne and Becker's muscular dystrophy have deletions of coding sequences in the dystrophin gene as shown by hybridisation with complementary DNA probes. This not only confirms the clinical diagnosis, which can be difficult in mild, sporadic cases, but also provides a definitive prenatal diagnostic test in families in which an affected boy has a gene deletion. Chorionic villus sampling in pregnancies at risk allows fetal sexing to be performed by chromosomal and DNA analysis and in male fetuses the presence or absence of a deletion can be determined. This allows unaffected male pregnancies to continue to term, which was not possible when only fetal sexing was available. Different deletions are seen in different families, and patterns are emerging that correspond to the Duchenne and Becker's forms of muscular dystrophy; this helps to distinguish between the two disorders in sporadic cases in young boys. Deletions causing a frame shift completely disrupt dystrophin production or function and cause Duchenne muscular dystrophy whereas deletions that do not disrupt the reading frame allow a modified protein to be produced, resulting in the milder Becker's form.

A deletion in the dystrophin gene does not help to identify gene carriers as on autoradiography the bands corresponding to the normal gene on one X chromosome mask the presence of a deleted gene on the other. Dosage studies (determining whether one or two copies of the relevant exons are present) are not generally reliable enough to permit prediction. If a probe that detects a deletion in a family also, however, identifies an associated RFLP this can be used in determining carrier state, as shown by the autoradiograph opposite. DNA from the affected boy (lane A) shows no bands with probe p20, indicating a gene deletion. His mother (lane B) is heterozygous for the associated RFLP (one allele being present on each chromosome), indicating that neither of her X chromosomes carries this gene deletion in the cells studied. Her carrier risk is not, however, negligible as she may carry a germline mutation which would not be detected by analysing leucocyte DNA. The boy's sister (lane C) is also heterozygous for the RFLP (one band inherited from her father and the other from her mother), indicating that she has not inherited a deleted gene from her mother. An inherited mutation would be present in all somatic cells and heterozygosity for the RFLP in leucocyte DNA confirms that she is not a carrier.

DNA analysis in genetic disorders

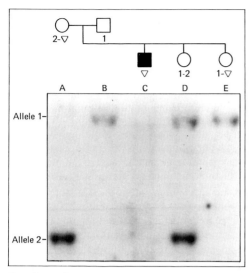

Restriction fragment length polymorphism and deletion detected with probe p20 in DNA digested with *Msp I* restriction endonuclease. (See text for interpretation.) ▽=Deletion.

Another example of deletion and RFLP analysis is shown in the autoradiograph opposite. The affected boy again has a gene deletion detected by probe p20 (lane C). His mother (lane A) is apparently homozygous for allele 2. One of the boy's sisters (lane E) has inherited an X chromosomal band from her father (lane B) but not her mother. The explanation of this apparent "non-maternity" is that the daughter has inherited a deleted gene from her mother, and this indicates that they are both carriers. The other sister (lane D) has inherited a paternal and a maternal band. The maternal band corresponds to the non-deleted gene, and this sister is therefore not a carrier.

DNA analysis has proved to be extremely valuable in investigating families with Duchenne and Becker's muscular dystrophy. Not only can many carriers be identified and offered definitive prenatal diagnosis but female relatives at low risk can commonly be identified and reassured. Several difficulties are still encountered: family studies are required and predictive tests may not be possible if the affected boy is no longer living; occasional families have uninformative DNA patterns with the currently available probes; and calculations are often complex. In sporadic cases the mother of an affected boy cannot be given a negligible risk because of the possibility of germline mosaicism, and even if population screening for carriers becomes possible the disorder will not be eradicated because of the frequency with which new mutations occur.

The autoradiograph of cystic fibrosis was reproduced by kind permission of Mr A Ivinson, that of the G8 haplotypes by Dr A Read, and that of Duchenne muscular dystrophy by Mr R Mountford, St Mary's Hospital, Manchester.

GLOSSARY

Alleles	Alternative forms of a gene or DNA sequence occurring at the same locus on homologous chromosomes.
Aneuploid	Chromosome number that is not an exact multiple of the haploid set—for example, 2n−1 or 2n+1.
Autoradiography	Detection of radiolabelled molecules with x ray film.
Autosome	Any chromosome other than the sex chromosomes.
Bayesian analysis	Mathematical method for calculating probability of carrier state in mendelian disorders by combining several independent likelihoods.
Carrier	Healthy person possessing a mutant gene in heterozygous form: also refers to a person with a balanced chromosomal translocation.
Chimaera	Presence in a person of two different cell lines derived from fusion of two zygotes.
Chorionic villus sampling	Procedure for obtaining fetally derived chorionic villus material for prenatal diagnosis.
Clone	All cells arising by mitotic division from a single original cell and having the same genetic constitution.
Codominant	Trait resulting from expression of both alleles at a particular locus in heterozygotes—for example, the ABO blood group system.
Codon	Coding sequence of three adjacent nucleotides.
Complementary DNA (cDNA)	Single stranded DNA synthesised from messenger RNA.
Concordance	Presence of the same trait in both members of a pair of twins.
Diploid	Normal state of human somatic cells, containing two haploid sets of chromosomes (2n).
Discordance	Presence of a trait in only one member of a pair of twins.
Dizygotic	Twins produced by the separate fertilisation of two different eggs.
DNA electrophoresis	Separation of DNA restriction fragments by electrophoresis in agarose gel.
DNA fingerprinting	Analysis that detects DNA pattern unique to a given person.
DNA polymerase	Enzyme concerned with synthesis of double stranded DNA from single stranded DNA.
Dominant	Trait expressed in people who are heterozygous for a particular gene.
Dysmorphology	Study of malformations arising from abnormal embryogenesis.
Embryo biopsy	Potential method for preimplantation diagnosis of genetic disorders used in conjunction with in vitro fertilisation.
Empirical risk	Risk of recurrence for multifactorial or polygenic disorders based on family studies.
Exon	Region of a gene transcribed into messenger RNA and translated into protein product.
Fetoscopy	Endoscopic procedure permitting direct visual examination of the fetus.
Genetic counselling	Process by which information on genetic disorders is given to a family.
Genome	Total DNA carried by a gamete.
Genotype	Genetic constitution of an individual person.
Gonadal mosaicism	Presence of a mutation in germline but not somatic cells, which results in transmission of a genetic disorder by a healthy person.
Haploid	Normal state of gametes, containing one set of chromosomes (n).
Haplotype	Particular set of alleles at closely linked loci on a single chromosome that are inherited together.
Hemizygote	Describes the genotype of males with an X linked trait, as males have only one X chromosome.
Heritability	The contribution of genetic as opposed to environmental factors to phenotypic variance.
Heterozygote	Person possessing different alleles at a particular locus on homologous chromosomes.
Holandric inheritance	Pattern of inheritance of genes on the Y chromosome.
Homologous chromosomes	Chromosomes that pair at meiosis and contain the same set of gene loci.
Homozygote	Person having two identical alleles at a particular locus on homologous chromosomes.
Hybridisation	Process by which single strands of DNA with homologous sequences bind together.
Intron	Region of a gene transcribed into messenger RNA but spliced out before translation into protein product.
Karyotype	Description of the chromosomes present in somatic cells.
Kilobase (kb)	1000 Base pairs (bp) of DNA.
Linkage	Term describing genes or DNA sequences situated close together on the same chromosome that tend to segregate together.
Linkage disequilibrium	Occurrence together of two particular linked alleles on the same chromosome more commonly than expected by chance.
Locus	Site of a specific gene or DNA sequence on a chromosome.
Lyonisation	Process of X chromosome inactivation in cells with more than one X chromosome.
Marker	General term for biochemical or DNA polymorphism occurring close to a gene and used in gene tracking.
Meiosis	Cell division during gametogenesis resulting in haploid gametes.
Mendelian disorder	Inherited disorder due to a defect in a single gene.
Mitosis	Cell division occurring in somatic cells resulting in diploid daughter cells.
Monosomy	Loss of one of a pair of homologous chromosomes.
Monozygotic	Twins derived from a single fertilised egg.
Mosaic	Presence in a person of two different cell lines derived from a single zygote.
Multifactorial inheritance	Disorder caused by interaction of more than one gene plus the effect of environment.
Multiple alleles	Existence of more than two alleles at a particular locus.
Mutation	Change in the structure of DNA.
Non-dysjunction	Failure of separation of paired chromosomes during cell division.
Obligate carrier	Family member who must be a heterozygous gene carrier, determined from the mode of inheritance and the pattern of affected relatives within the family.
Oligoprobe	A short DNA probe whose hybridisation is sensitive to a single base mismatch.
Oncogene	Gene with potential to cause cancer.
Penetrance	Probability that a disease genotype will result in an abnormal phenotype.
Phenotype	Physical or biochemical characteristics of a person reflecting genetic constitution and environmental influence.
Point mutation	Substitution of a single base pair in DNA molecule that may affect protein synthesis.
Polygenic inheritance	Disorder caused by interaction between more than one gene.
Polymerase chain reaction	Method of amplification of specific DNA sequences by repeated cycles of DNA synthesis to permit rapid analysis of DNA restriction fragments subsequently.
Polymorphism	Genetic characteristic with more than one common form in a population.
Polyploid	Chromosome numbers representing multiples of

57

Glossary

the haploid set greater than diploid—for example, 3n.

Polysome Group of ribosomes associated with a particular messenger RNA molecule.

Post-translational modification Alterations to protein structure after synthesis.

Proband Index case through which a family is identified.

Probe Radiolabelled DNA fragment used to detect complementary sequences in DNA sample.

Pseudogene Functionless copy of a known gene.

Pulse field gel electrophoresis Method for separating large fragments of DNA (50-10 000 kb) by altering the direction of the electrical field during electrophoresis.

Purine Nitrogenous base: adenine or guanine.

Pyrimidine Nitrogenous base: cytosine, thymine, or uracil.

Recessive Trait expressed in people who are homozygous or hemizygous for a particular gene but not in those who are heterozygous for the gene.

Recombination Crossing over between homologous chromosomes at meiosis which separates linked loci.

Restriction endonuclease Enzyme that cleaves double stranded DNA at a specific sequence.

Restriction fragments DNA fragments produced by restriction endonuclease digestion of sample DNA.

Restriction fragment length polymorphism (RFLP) Variation in size of DNA fragments produced by restriction endonuclease digestion due to variation in DNA sequence at the enzyme recognition site.

Reverse transcriptase Enzyme catalysing the synthesis of complementary DNA from messenger RNA.

Segregation Separation of alleles during meiosis so that each gamete contains only one member of each pair of alleles.

Southern blotting Process of transferring DNA fragments from agarose gel on to nitrocellulose filter or nylon membrane.

Splicing Removal of introns and joining of exons in messenger RNA.

Trait Recognisable phenotype due to a genetic character.

Transcription Production of messenger RNA from DNA sequence in gene.

Translation Production of protein from messenger RNA sequence.

Translocation Transfer of chromosomal material between two non-homologous chromosomes.

Triploid Cells containing three haploid sets of chromosomes (3n).

Trisomy Cells containing one more than the normal diploid set of chromosomes (2n+1).

Unifactorial Inheritance controlled by single gene pair.

SUPPORT GROUPS

There are support groups for families with many different genetic disorders. The following is intended as a guide and does not include all existing self help groups.

Association to Combat Huntington's Chorea
(COMBAT)
Borough House
34a Station Road
Hinckley
Leicestershire LE10 1AP

Association for Research into Restricted
Growth
24 Pinchfield
Maple Cross
Rickmansworth
Hertfordshire

Association for Spina Bifida and
Hydrocephalus
Tavistock House North
Tavistock Square
London WC1H 9HJ

The Arthrogryposis Group (TAG)
Lawrence Robinson
27 Melksham Close
Macclesfield
Cheshire SK11 8NH

The British Retinitis Pigmentosa Society
24 Palmer Close
Redhill
Surrey RH1 4BX

Brittle Bone Society
122 City Road
Dundee DD2 2PW

Cleft Lip and Palate Association
Dental Department
Hospital for Sick Children
Great Ormond Street
London WC1N 3JH

The Cystic Fibrosis Research Trust
5 Blyth Road
Bromley
Kent BR1 3RS

Down's Children's Association
4 Oxford Street
London W1

Dystrophic Epidermolysis Bullosa Research
Association (DEBRA)
Suite 4, 1st Floor
1 Kings Road
Crowthorne
Berkshire RH11 7BG

The Friedreich's Ataxia Group
The Common
Cranleigh
Surrey GU6 8SB

The Foundation for the Study of Infant
Deaths
5th Floor
4 Grosvenor Place
London SW1X 7HD

The Haemophilia Society
PO Box 9
16 Trinity Street
London SE1 1DE

The Neurofibromatosis Association (LINK)
1 The Alders
Hanworth
Middlesex TW13 6NU

Muscular Dystrophy Group of Great Britain
26 Borough High Street
London SE1 9QG

Marfan Association
Cardiovascular Pathology
Jenner Wing
St Georges Hospital Medical School
Tooting
London SW17 0RE

National Deaf Children's Society
31 Gloucester Place
London W1 4EA

National Federation of the Blind of the UK
20 Cannon Close
Raynes Park
London SW20

National Society for Phenylketonuria and
Allied Disorders
18 Wood Close
Joydens Wood
Bexley
Kent

Research Trust for Metabolic Diseases in
Children
53 Beam Street
Nantwich
Cheshire CW5 5NF

Royal National Institute for the Blind
224 Great Portland Street
London W1N 6AA

Royal National Institute for the Deaf
105 Gower Street
London WC1E 6AH

Sickle Cell Society
c/o Brent Community Health Council
16 High Street
Harlesden
London NW10 4XL

The Society for Mucopolysaccharide
Diseases
30 Westwood Drive
Little Chalfont
Buckinghamshire

UK Thalassaemia Society
107 Nightingale Lane
London N8 7QY

Tuberous Sclerosis Association of Great
Britain
Little Barnsley Farm
Milton Road
Catshill
Bromsgrove
Worcestershire B61 0WQ

Tay-Sachs and Allied Diseases Association
17 Sydney Road
Barkingside
Ilford
Essex IG5 2ED

INDEX

Index